Working with Survivors
of Sibling Sexual Abuse

from the author

We Are Still Here
What Counsellors and Therapists Can Learn from the
Lived Experiences of Child Sexual Abuse Survivors
Christiane Sanderson
Foreword by Fay Maxted
ISBN 978 1 78592 232 9
eISBN 978 1 78450 511 0

Counselling Skills for Working with Shame
Christiane Sanderson
ISBN 978 1 84905 562 8
eISBN 978 1 78450 001 6

Counselling Skills for Working with Trauma
Healing from Child Sexual Abuse, Sexual Violence and Domestic Abuse
Christiane Sanderson
ISBN 978 1 84905 326 6
eISBN 978 0 85700 743 8

Counselling Adult Survivors of Child Sexual Abuse
Third Edition
Christiane Sanderson
ISBN 978 1 84310 335 6
eISBN 978 1 84642 532 5

WORKING with SURVIVORS of SIBLING SEXUAL ABUSE

A Guide to Therapeutic Support and Protection for Children and Adults

Christiane Sanderson
Foreword by Simon Hackett

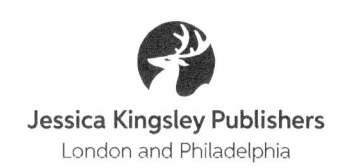

Jessica Kingsley Publishers
London and Philadelphia

First published in Great Britain in 2024 by Jessica Kingsley Publishers
An imprint of John Murray Press

1

Copyright © Christiane Sanderson 2024

The right of Christiane Sanderson to be identified as the Author of the Work has been asserted by her in accordance with the Copyright, Designs and Patents Act 1988.

Foreword © Simon Hackett 2024

All rights reserved. No part of this publication may be reproduced, stored in a retrieval system, or transmitted, in any form or by any means without the prior written permission of the publisher, nor be otherwise circulated in any form of binding or cover other than that in which it is published and without a similar condition being imposed on the subsequent purchaser.

A CIP catalogue record for this title is available from the British Library and the Library of Congress

ISBN 978 1 80501 126 2
eISBN 978 1 80501 127 9

Printed and bound in Great Britain by CPI Group

Jessica Kingsley Publishers' policy is to use papers that are natural, renewable and recyclable products and made from wood grown in sustainable forests. The logging and manufacturing processes are expected to conform to the environmental regulations of the country of origin.

Jessica Kingsley Publishers
Carmelite House
50 Victoria Embankment
London EC4Y 0DZ

www.jkp.com

John Murray Press
Part of Hodder & Stoughton Ltd
An Hachette Company

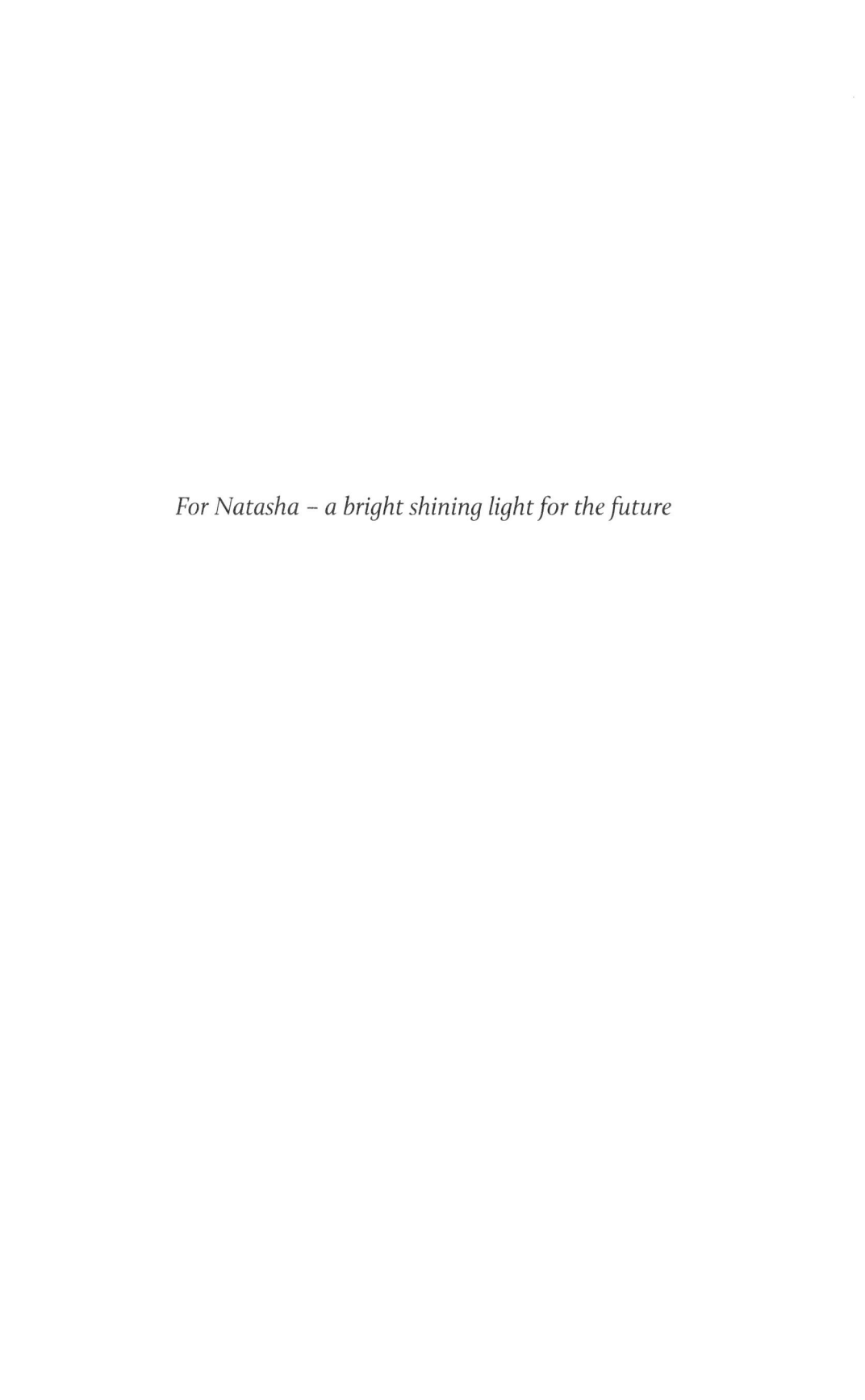

For Natasha – a bright shining light for the future

Contents

	Foreword by Professor Simon Hackett	8
	Acknowledgements	11
	Preface	13
	Introduction	17
1.	The Nature of Sibling Sexual Abuse	33
2.	Risk Factors in Sibling Sexual Abuse	45
3.	Typical Sexual Development and Sexual Behaviour in Children and Young People	57
4.	Atypical Sexual Behaviour in Children and Young People	68
5.	The Impact of Sibling Sexual Abuse	81
6.	Understanding the Sexually Abused Child	95
7.	The Long-Term Effects of Sibling Sexual Abuse on Adult Survivors	115
8.	The Intrapersonal and Relational Effects of Sibling Sexual Abuse in Adult Survivors	132
9.	Working with Adult Survivors of Sibling Sexual Abuse: Trauma-Informed Practice	142
10.	Working with Adult Survivors of Sibling Sexual Abuse: The Therapeutic Relationship	165
11.	The Prevention of Sibling Sexual Abuse	180
12.	Future Research and Professional Practice	195
	References	202
	Resources	210
	Subject Index	218
	Author Index	222

Foreword

PROFESSOR SIMON HACKETT

We have learnt a lot about child sexual abuse over the last two decades.

In no small part, this increased awareness has come about as a result of the enormous courage and bravery shown by survivors of abuse who have come forward, often at great personal cost, to share their childhood experiences of hurt and harm.

As I write the foreword to this book, the Independent Inquiry into Child Sexual Abuse (IICSA) has just published its final report after seven years of investigation into sexual abuse across a wide variety of settings in England and Wales (Jay et al., 2022). In both its final report and its 19 interim reports, IICSA casts a critical light onto the nature and contexts of sexual harm affecting children *outside of the home*.

Yet as part of its Truth Project, IICSA also heard testimony from more than 6,200 victims and survivors, many of whom talked about having been sexually abused *at home*, usually by a known and trusted family member. For some, it was the first time they had ever spoken about their abuse. For others who had been able to report what was happening to them as children, their accounts were often ignored or not taken seriously.

Similarly, a 2015 report into child sexual abuse in the family environment by the Office of the Children's Commissioner for England (2015) estimated that only 1 in 8 sexually abused children are ever identified by professionals. This report argued that the scale of sexual abuse in the family environment is such that it needs to be acknowledged as a national priority.

Alongside these insights, we have also had to challenge orthodox assumptions about who is responsible for child sexual abuse. We now know that a high proportion of all sexually abusive behaviour is displayed by other young people under the age of 18, not just adults. Indeed, it has become something of a truism that between a quarter and a third of all sexual abuse coming to the attention of professionals relates to children as the alleged perpetrator. The figure may be much higher; recent data trends suggest that up to half of all reports of sexual crime made to police involve children as the alleged offenders.

Given the frequency by which sexual abuse occurs in family settings *and* the significant proportion of sexual abuse committed by young people, it is surprising, then, that so little has been written about sibling sexual abuse. It is a subject that has been neglected in research, in policy, and in the media. As the title of this book suggests, it remains a taboo subject. There is no doubt that sibling sexual abuse is a very significant social and public health issue that affects the lives of very many children and adults. According to Yates and Allardyce (2021), sibling sexual abuse is likely to be the most common form of intra-familial sexual abuse, estimated to be up to three times as common as sexual abuse by a parent.

Although sibling abuse shares many of the same characteristics of other types of child sexual abuse, characterised as it often is by secrecy, shame, and guilt, it also presents some specific complexities and challenges. For example, I remember a couple talking to me about the shock and absolute pain of finding out that their older son had been sexually abusing their younger son. They didn't know how or whether they could balance their love and concern for both of their children. They said it was like a bomb had gone off in their family, destroying it, and they didn't know how they could ever rebuild it.

In a research study I was involved in, adults who had experienced or perpetrated sibling sexual abuse many years ago told me that it had never been properly addressed or even discussed with their siblings or parents after the siblings had become adults. The sibling sexual abuse remained, for many, like an open wound that nobody had sought to help them to heal.

This book therefore is both urgently needed and timely. Its author, Christiane Sanderson, writes with clarity about a complex topic, carefully presenting the evidence and writing sensitively, empathically, and practically about what can be done to address sibling sexual abuse. The book is remarkable in its ability to speak to survivors, professionals, and parents alike. Few authors have attempted, let alone achieved, this. Christiane throws off the veil of secrecy associated with sibling sexual abuse, helps raise our awareness of this issue as a professional community, and gives hope to survivors that they will be heard.

Professor Simon Hackett
Durham University, October 2022

References

Jay, A., Evans, M., Frank, I., & Sharpling, D. (2022). *The report of the independent inquiry into child sexual abuse*. IICSA.

Office of the Children's Commissioner for England (2015). *Protecting children from harm: A critical assessment of child sexual abuse in the family network in England and priorities for action*. Office of the Children's Commissioner for England.

Yates, P., & Allardyce, S. (2021). *Sibling sexual abuse: A knowledge and practice overview*. CSA Centre.

Acknowledgements

My thanks go to all survivors of sibling sexual abuse who have shown enormous courage to give voice to their experiences. It has been an honour to bear witness and accompany them on their journey.

The book would not have come to fruition without the unstinting support of Stephen Jones at Jessica Kingsley Publishers. I thank him for recognising the importance of raising awareness about the hidden nature of sibling sexual abuse, its impact, and how practitioners can best support adult survivors. Thank you too to to Pauli Roos and Emma Holak for their editorial support and sage advice.

Finally, I could not have written this book without the unwavering support of my colleagues Dr Jo-Ann Cruywagen, Nicole Proia, Dr Emma Kay, Professor Anna Seymour, Professor Mick Cooper, Linda Dominguez MBE and all the staff at One in Four. In addition, I would like to thank Ravi Kumar for believing in this book, Professor Simon Hackett for his wisdom, and Fleur Strong for her energy, My gratitude as always goes to James, Max and Lucy who held and sustained me throughout this journey.

These things happen between brother and sister

This is how I was dismissed when I tried to disclose
the abuse by my brother the second time.
The first time I tried to disclose 18 years after it happened the person
said to me 'don't make this into something bigger than it is'.
By this point I had barely said one sentence but what it
had included was my brother was 12 and I was 10 years
old, that was enough for that person to dismiss me.
These kinds of off-hand dismissive,
judgemental comments shut me up.
Made me feel small.
Amplified the shame, confusion, and isolation
I was already feeling inside.
That first time shut me up for another 6 years.
The second time thankfully I was able to open my mouth later
and challenge what was said and was well received. But that's
because I had spent time building up my internal resources.
These comments, dismissive and judgemental, are dangerous and just
intensify those feelings inside that we are wrong or bad in some way.
I would ask that all professionals – listen – hear what is
being said to you without judgement. Hear the feelings,
the experiences, the thoughts of that person. Hear
and listen to what they are trying to tell you.
Do not judge.
All I would have wanted was someone to
do that. To listen. To say to me:
'I hear you'.
It took another 8 years before I was able to reach out again.
Another 8 years of holding onto the shame, confusion,
and hopelessness, by this time I was in my 40s.
This time thankfully I was received without judgement,
I was heard and the abuse that happened was validated.

Anonymous

Preface

Sibling relationships have traditionally been viewed as generally benign, nurturing, and developmentally growth promoting. Many children value and appreciate their siblings and experience them as protective attachment figures, who act as a buffer between them and their parents, are fun playmates, wise teachers, and provide support in childhood and throughout adulthood. Healthy sibling relationships have also been shown to shape siblings' sense of self, self-identity, and self-esteem, as well as promoting relational worth, developing relationship skills, mentalisation, empathy, mutuality, and how to compromise (White & Hughes, 2018), all of which aid positive psychosocial functioning.

Conversely, sibling relationships can also be competitive and full of rivalry, hostility, combative, and conflict ridden, wherein ferocious arguing, bullying, and scapegoating is normalised (White & Hughes, 2018). The true nature of sibling relationships is that they can fluctuate and change over time and can contain aspects of healthy relational dynamics as well as competitive ones (Yates & Allardyce, 2021), which can make it hard to differentiate at what point teasing or banter becomes bullying, when quarrelling becomes hostile, aggressive, and harmful, or when play fighting becomes violent or abusive.

While the majority of sibling relationships are positive, there are some that are unsafe or abusive due to subtle or unacknowledged power imbalances such as gender, age, birth order, cognitive ability, dependency needs, or cultural norms and expectations. Favoured children may be accorded extra power and privileged status, making it impossible for siblings to challenge them, while older children who are given authority when in loco parentis and left in charge of younger siblings may misuse their power (Punch, 2008).

The complexity of sibling relationships and the potential for abusive sibling interaction has been under-researched and under-represented in the child protection and therapeutic literature. This is in part due to a lack of recognition of power imbalances, and because sibling interactions are more hidden as they often spend prolonged periods of time together without parental supervision, wherein interactions and boundaries become unfettered and unregulated. This can lead to expressions of anger and hostility, along with threats of and actual physical violence, as well as sexual abuse, which younger or less powerful siblings may be too terrified to reveal for fear of not being believed, or punished.

Safe sibling relationships are invaluable for younger siblings to express their curiosity about themselves, others, and the world, including their sexual curiosity. While some sexual interactions between young siblings are consensual and consist of sexual play and experimentation, some are non-consensual, harmful, and abusive and should not be minimised or dismissed as harmless. To mitigate confusion it is essential that parents and professionals have a clearer understanding of what constitutes sibling sexual abuse (SSA), and what is considered to be developmentally typical sexual behaviour between siblings, and what is considered to be problematic or harmful sexual behaviour (HSB).

As there is currently no universally agreed definition of SSA, it remains under-reported and under-recorded by authorities, and will remain so unless SSA is acknowledged and accorded a separate category rather than being subsumed under child sexual abuse (CSA). Despite the hidden nature of SSA, it is estimated that it is up to three times more prevalent than intergenerational sexual abuse perpetrated by parents, and equally harmful. Research has shown that SSA commonly involves an older brother abusing a younger sister, although there is evidence of brother to brother, sister to sister, and sister to brother SSA, as well as more than one sibling abusing single or multiple younger siblings.

Some siblings who commit SSA may themselves have a history of CSA or SSA and as a result have 'dual status' in being both a victim of sexual abuse and engaging in HSB, and needing to have access to specialist therapeutic support as well as being held accountable for the harm they have caused. This needs to extend to appropriate support during adulthood in order to manage any dissonance between having committed SSA as a child and their sense of self as an adult, especially as they become parents themselves. Professionals need to be mindful that the majority of children who commit SSA do not go on to perpetrate sexual abuse in adulthood and should not be treated as 'mini-adult offenders', and that they need to respond proportionally to ensure such assumptions do not contaminate safeguarding assessments in adulthood.

The risk of committing or experiencing SSA arises out of the complex interplay of a number of factors such as individual predispositions, neurodivergence, a history of sexual abuse, trauma, or adverse childhood experiences, family dynamics, and socio-cultural factors. In addition, the digitisation of sex and early exposure to pornography can lead to re-enactments of sexual behaviour with younger siblings. While the relative contribution of each of these factors is still unclear, further research could illuminate this. In raising awareness of the nature of SSA and its impact professionals will be more adequately resourced to respond to and support children, families, siblings, and adult survivors, and develop appropriate interventions and preventive strategies.

The confusion, shame, and secrecy inherent in SSA makes it extremely difficult for children and adult survivors to disclose, and for families to seek support as they fear being blamed or judged. To remove the taboo of SSA it is crucial that all those in the child's psychosocial world, including professionals, are aware of the risk of SSA, the motivations to commit SSA, as well as the impact on the child and later adult, so that they can enable survivors to give voice to their lived experience and the quality of their relationship with their siblings, without judgement or imposing their own views or assumptions around sibling sexual interactions.

As SSA occurs within family settings it is essential that professionals have an understanding of diverse family identities and systems, as well as family dynamics that may elevate the risk of HSB. Assessments need to focus on risk of harm, and the impact on the siblings involved in SSA, as well as parents and other siblings, and the risk of suicidal ideation in either of the siblings. In order to support children and adults who have experienced SSA, professionals need to be aware of the impact of SSA and recognise that while there may be no overt signs of harm at the time, there may be delayed trauma reactions in adolescence or adulthood. Many children who experience SSA do not necessarily see this as abusive or harmful at the time, and may not do so until adulthood when they enter intimate relationships or have their own children. Professionals need to be aware of such delayed trauma and respond appropriately rather than minimise the harm done.

To support and help survivors of SSA to recover and heal from their experiences, mental health professionals and practitioners need to be aware of the complexity of SSA and adopt a relational and strengths-based approach, which incorporates the fundamental principles of trauma-informed practice and the Power Threat Meaning Framework (Johnstone & Boyle, 2018). This needs to be combined with a phased oriented approach to titrate exposure to the SSA experiences and conducted in the presence of a warm, compassionate, and genuinely caring relationship, where survivors can learn new ways of relating to others and develop relationship skills.

My hope is that this book, in unveiling the taboo and hidden nature of SSA, and enhancing awareness of its impact on children and adult survivors, will enable parents and professionals to acknowledge the harmful effects of SSA, and enable survivors to give voice to their lived experience safe in the knowledge that they will be heard and believed rather than dismissed.

Christiane Sanderson

Introduction

It is estimated that one-third of sexual abuse is perpetrated by children, with some as young as four engaging in harmful sexual behaviour (HSB). Overt peer-to-peer abuse is commonly seen in sexual harassment and sexual bullying, peer-to-peer sexual exploitation, and the use of sexual violence and rape in gangs. There is however a more nuanced, often unspoken type of HSB which is usually under-reported as it masquerades as consensual sexual experimentation between children, especially siblings, step-siblings, and cousins (Sanderson, 2004; Yates & Allardyce, 2021).

To fully differentiate between consensual sexual experimentation and sexually harmful behaviour it is critical to understand both developmentally typical and atypical sexual interactions in children and young people. This book will examine the nature and dynamics of sibling sexual abuse (SSA), its impact and long-term effects. It will distinguish between typical age appropriate consensual sexual curiosity and sexual experimentation and atypical sexual behaviour which is non-consensual and sexually harmful.

There has been an increase in the reporting of HSB with an estimated one-third of child sexual abuse (CSA) committed by children, with some as young as four engaging in HSB. Overt peer-on-peer abuse is commonly seen in sexual harassment, sexual bullying, peer-on-peer sexual exploitation, rape in gang culture, and the use of sexual violence and rape among young people. The degree of sexual violence, especially against females, is captured on the *everyone's invited* website which has exposed the extent of rape culture both in schools and the wider community.

There is a more hidden form of child-on-child abuse which is unspoken, under-disclosed, under-reported, and under-recorded (Carlson et al., 2006). It is estimated that SSA is three times more common than intergenerational CSA (Wiehe, 1997; Krienert & Walsh, 2011; Stroebel et al., 2013; Caffaro & Conn-Caffaro, 2014), and that between a quarter to half of HSB involves siblings or close family relatives such as cousins, half cousins, step-siblings, half-siblings, or adoptive siblings (Shaw et al., 2000; Hardy, 2001; Beckett, 2006; Atwood, 2007; Finkelhor, 2009; Hackett, 2014; Hackett et al., 2019). Despite the extent of SSA it is often overlooked or minimised by parents and professionals as it is seen as developmentally normal, consensual sexual exploration and deemed as less harmful than intergenerational CSA (Yates & Allardyce, 2021).

The failure to recognise HSB and SSA is in part due to a lack of knowledge and awareness of SSA as it is under-researched (Tener et al., 2017), and the belief that sexual activity between siblings serves a developmental function to satisfy sexual curiosity and is inevitable in families, and thus in essence harmless (Friedrich et al., 1998). The lack of research prevents parents and professionals from fully understanding the nature and dynamics intrinsic in SSA, its impact and long-term effects. As a result sexual activity between siblings is often minimised, normalised, or dismissed, leaving the child and later survivor in a state of confusion and doubt about what happened to them.

Definition

Currently there is no clear, agreed definition of what constitutes SSA, making it difficult not only for survivors to know whether their sexual experience counts as sexual abuse, but also professionals such as the police, children's services, and practitioners working with children or adult survivors. In addition, the absence of a clear definition means it is harder to report or record it, as authorities often subsume SSA under the general category of CSA.

In the UK, sibling sexual abuse is currently subsumed under the general definition of child sexual abuse, which is defined as behaviour that:

> involves forcing or enticing a child or young person to take part in sexual activities, not necessarily involving a high level of violence, whether or not the child is aware of what is happening. The activities may involve physical contact, including assault by penetration (for example, rape or oral sex) or non-penetrative acts such as masturbation, kissing, rubbing and touching outside of clothing. They may also include non-contact

activities, such as involving children in looking at, or in the production of, sexual images, watching sexual activities, encouraging children to behave in sexually inappropriate ways, or grooming a child in preparation for abuse. Sexual abuse can take place online, and technology can be used to facilitate offline abuse. Sexual abuse is not solely perpetrated by adult males. Women can also commit acts of sexual abuse, as can other children. (Department for Education, 2018, p. 103)

Yates and Allardyce (2021) propose that SSA generally refers to children who grow up in the same family whether they are biological siblings, step-siblings, half-siblings, foster siblings, or adopted siblings, and can be committed by both male and female children. McCartan et al. (2021, p. 6) proposed a working definition for SSA in their research for Rape Crisis England Wales as 'any form of sexualized behaviour or action, contact and non-contact, between siblings when they were under the age of 18'.

Research indicates that while the most common form of SSA is committed by brother to sister (Caffaro & Conn-Caffaro, 1998), it can also occur from brother to brother, sister to sister, or sister to brother, and be committed by more than one sibling against one or multiple siblings (Yates & Allardyce, 2021). A compelling finding in McCartan et al.'s (2021) research is that 28% of the SSA committed in their study was by sisters and not brothers, which suggests that SSA is not necessarily a gendered form of abuse, and that parents and professionals must be open-minded with regard to who commits SSA.

In some cases of SSA the sibling who has harmed may have 'dual status' in having been sexually abused and committing SSA. While some siblings who have been sexually abused go on to commit HSB, this does not predict HSB or SSA (Stripe & Stermac, 2003; Stathopoulos, 2012) as the majority of people who have been sexually abused do not go on to sexually abuse. Professionals must guard against making such assumptions (Glaser, 1991; Wiehe, 1998; Caspi, 2011; McCartan et al., 2021; Yates & Allardyce, 2021) to avoid stigmatisation.

Professionals' beliefs about the nature of sibling relationships can result in ignoring or minimising power differentials such as age, gender, privilege, status, or cultural norms and expectations. In addition, many parents and professionals find it difficult to acknowledge sexual development in children and find it less threatening to view children as sexually naïve or innocent than believe that children are capable of sexually harming other children. This is exacerbated by views of children's sexual curiosity, and sexual play and experimentation between siblings being normalised, especially when there are no initial clear signs of harm (Allardyce & Yates, 2018).

Research on the nature of sibling relationships and how these impact and shape attachments and future relationships has been limited as traditionally the emphasis has been on the centrality of the parent–child relationship. As a result many psychotherapeutic models have largely ignored the effect of sibling relationships on attachment and later mental health, and are coloured by the assumption that sibling relationships are inherently non-abusive and primarily positive, and developmentally nurturing (Yates & Allardyce, 2021). Much of the literature focuses on the positive aspects of sibling relationships rather than more negative aspects such as physical abuse (interpreted as play fighting), humiliation and shaming (interpreted as teasing), or sexual abuse (seen as normative sexual play and experimentation). While there is an acknowledgement that siblings argue and fight, generally speaking sibling relationships are perceived as being based on inherent mutual alliances, and thus more equal with little or no power differential (Yates & Allardyce, 2021). The emphasis has been on growth-promoting aspects and protective factors that act as a buffer against parental discipline.

McCartan et al. (2021) also found that some professionals were not aware of the complexity and nuances of SSA, and either minimised these or felt overwhelmed by any form of sexual behaviour between siblings including developmentally normal and exploratory sexual behaviour. They reported that it was 'less harmful than other kinds of abuse', or saw it as 'normal sexual exploration that maybe went a little too far', or found it 'inevitable, given the dynamics in the family'. Given the disparity of professional reactions, professionals need to be mindful that this can lead to multi-agency disagreements about risk and harm.

The Nature of SSA

The range of sexual behaviour between siblings ranges from normative, developmental sexual curiosity, consensual sexual play through to non-consensual sexual experimentation, HSB, sexual assault, and rape. Given the spectrum of SSA it includes both non-contact and contact sexual activities including coercing a sibling to look at sexual images, including pornography, or sexually explicit films, watching the sibling undress or while going to the lavatory or bathing, or forcing them to engage in HSB with other children (Yates & Allardyce, 2021). Contact SSA includes the full range of non-consensual sexual touching, stroking, kissing, licking, as well as oral, vaginal, or anal penetration. These sexual activities are rarely a one-off incident and can persist for long periods of time, sometimes years during which the HSB can escalate and intensify (Katz & Hamama, 2017).

The complex and subtle nature of SSA makes it hard for siblings to recognise that it is HSB, especially if they have been enticed into the sexual activities through playing a game, or feeling complicit in the activity. As they enjoy extra attention from an older sibling and enjoy playing games with him or her, they feel that the sexual activity is just another game rather than abuse. In addition, they are often not aware that they are being groomed, or that the sibling who has harmed is exerting power and control over them. In some cases the sibling who has harmed will terrorise the sibling who is being harmed through the use of emotional abuse, humiliation, or physical violence, which renders them silent and unable to speak the unspeakable.

In the absence of penetration and physical violence, many children do not see themselves as having been subjected to sexual abuse until late adolescence or adulthood when they become sexually active and experience delayed trauma reactions (Enns et al., 1995; Ballantine, 2012), or enter therapy for unexplained trauma reactions. This attests to the need for psychoeducation on the harmful nature of SSA.

It is essential that professionals recognise that children and adult survivors of SSA are not homogeneous, nor are the children who commit SSA. There are a range of motivations that underpin HSB and SSA and professionals need to be aware of these to fully understand the specific dynamics in each individual case. Research has shown that the vulnerability to committing SSA is predicated on the complex interplay of individual factors in the child, neurodivergence, exposure to trauma and adverse childhood experiences (ACEs), family dynamics and socio-cultural factors such as gendered cultural beliefs and ideologies, racism, socio-economic status, religion, the premature sexualisation of children, early exposure to pornography, and marginalisation (McCartan et al., 2021). Professionals need to be mindful of how these intersect and shape the child's environment and impact on the risk of committing SSA. Given the role of family dynamics and socio-cultural factors, professionals need to be mindful of the ripple effect of SSA and not just its impact on the sibling who is being harmed and the sibling who has harmed; they also need to take into consideration the impact on other family members.

Developmentally Typical Sexual Behaviour versus Developmentally Atypical Sexual Behaviour

In order to prevent the normalisation and minimisation of SSA it is crucial to distinguish between consensual sexual experimentation and HSB and to understand the difference between what is generally considered to be developmentally typical and atypical psychosexual development in children and young people. This allows for greater awareness of what is age appropriate, consensual sexual curiosity and experimentation, and what is atypical sexual behaviour which is non-consensual and harmful.

Children who experience SSA or who commit SSA are not a homogeneous group and professionals need to be aware of the range of motivations that underpin sexual behaviour between siblings, which can range from normative consensual sexual play and sexual experimentation to the assertion of power and control, to non-consensual HSB and rape (see Chapters 3 and 4). The spectrum of motivation associated with SSA can range from sexual curiosity, to huddling together for protection, safety, and soothing, which becomes sexualised, to sexual satisfaction, gaining mastery over their own CSA, to jealousy, anger, rage, and hostility (see Chapter 4). Given this broad range of motivations, it is important to recognise gender and power and control dynamics in which older, bigger, stronger, or more powerful siblings coerce, threaten, or manipulate younger, less powerful siblings into engaging in non-consensual and inappropriate sexual activity.

Research has shown that SSA can occur in any family and is shaped by multiple factors and the interplay of individual and systemic factors, as well as cultural and psychosocial factors (Caffaro, 2020; McCartan et al., 2021). These include the child's individual predisposition, exposure to trauma and ACEs as well as family dynamics such as physical and emotional availability of parents, quality of attachment, setting of clear physical and sexual boundaries, supervision, and appropriate interventions. Family identities and family functioning are further influenced by socio-cultural factors such as race, discrimination and marginalisation, socio-economic status, religion, cultural norms and expectations, and exposure to pornography and how these intersect (see Chapter 2).

What is not clear is the relative contribution of each of the factors, and it is imperative that professionals do not ascribe responsibility to any one particular factor to the exclusion of others. This is critical as all the factors need to be examined and assessed on a case-by-case basis to see how they correlate and lead to an increased risk of committing SSA. Professionals need to guard against focusing on one single causal factor to ensure that they do not direct fault and blame on either the child or the parents and dysfunctional family dynamics, or cultural norms.

The subtlety of SSA and its normalisation means that not all children experience it as abusive or traumatic at the time it occurs. As there is huge variation in terms of impact, long-term effects, and outcome of SSA, professionals need to be mindful of not making simplistic assumptions. Generally speaking long-term effects include dissociation and trauma reactions, difficulties in relationships, fear of intimacy, compromised sexuality, chronic shame, and changed perceptions of the self. Many survivors of SSA and CSA perceive relationships as dangerous, including the therapeutic relationship, and will find it hard to engage in these if they feel they are not heard or the SSA is minimised or dismissed (McCartan et al., 2021; Yates & Allardyce, 2022).

In essence when working with children or adult survivors of SSA, no one size fits all and practitioners need to be able to cultivate flexibility in their thinking and not be too prescriptive in their interventions. What might work for one child or adult survivor may not be appropriate for another, and may be detrimental (see Chapters 9 and 10).

Disclosure

The impact of SSA does not end when the SSA ends but can be exacerbated during disclosure and in some cases can lead to re-traumatisation and post-disclosure trauma. Disclosure of SSA can be very difficult for both children and adult survivors for myriad reasons as they fear not being believed, judged or blamed, or punished. A palpable fear is how parents will react to the disclosure and that it might be minimised or that they will not intervene or stop the abuse, and that it might escalate. The fear of disclosure is intensified if the sibling who is being harmed feels complicit in the abuse or feels ashamed for becoming sexually aroused (Caffaro & Conn-Caffaro, 2014; O'Keefe et al., 2014) and that they will be held responsible for the SSA rather than legitimising it as abuse.

A further fear is how the disclosure will impact on the family and create conflict and split loyalties, fragmentation, or disintegration of the family. In addition, many siblings who are being harmed want to protect their sibling and do not want him or her to get into trouble. The wish to preserve the family is a powerful barrier to disclosure with some children suffering in silence and not being able to give voice to SSA until late adulthood (McCartan et al., 2021; Yates & Allardyce, 2021). Disclosure either in childhood or later in adulthood can elicit suicidal ideation in the sibling who is being harmed as the trauma is reactivated, or in the sibling who has harmed due to shame, guilt, or the dissonance between SSA committed in childhood and the adult sense of self, especially if they have children and safeguarding concerns are triggered.

Parents may also fear disclosure as they may not understand where the line is between developmentally normal sexual curiosity and SSA, and are unsure of how to respond or what to do, especially if they themselves were sexually abused in childhood, or committed SSA (Yates & Allardyce, 2021). They often fear involving the authorities in case either sibling is removed from the family and taken into care, or that the sibling who has harmed is sent to a youth offending institution. They will also fear being judged or blamed for the SSA or made to feel ashamed.

Parents often feel powerless and overwhelmed in the face of revelations of SSA and feel that they have failed both of their children, and feel helpless with regard to managing the disclosure or how to access support. They may also be suffused with unbearable levels of anger towards the sibling who has disclosed, the sibling who has harmed, and the professionals involved, and uncertain which sibling to support. In addition, disclosure can activate powerful feelings of loss and grief, as well as fears of stigmatisation and isolation (Yates & Allardyce, 2021).

While parental responses to disclosure can vary enormously, they are central in promoting better outcomes with regard to mental health and the resolution of trauma (Caffaro, 2020; Yates & Allardyce, 2022). While some parents are able to be supportive of both siblings, some struggle with denial, have split loyalties in which sibling to believe and support, or blame each other for allowing the SSA to happen (Yates & Allardyce, 2021). If a parent has experienced CSA themselves they may become overwhelmed by returning memories of their own abuse. Professionals need to be aware that the initial denial of the SSA does not mean that parents will not seek out support, nor does it mean that parents who have sought support will necessarily engage in any proposed interventions (Yates & Allardyce, 2021).

Like the sibling who is being harmed, parents will fear the ripple effect of the disclosure on the whole family with regard to split loyalties, the impact on the siblings not abused, and confusing feelings around the sibling who has harmed and anger towards the sibling who is being harmed for disclosing and breaking up the family.

The uncertainty and confusion about whether it is SSA significantly affects the disclosure and reporting of the HSB, as does the parental response. Parents who are attentive and listen to the child, validate his or her experience and seek professional support for both the sibling who is being harmed and the sibling who has harmed, and support the siblings can help enormously in facilitating healing and reparation and work towards keeping the family intact and the sibling who is being harmed safe. Parental responses that are negative and do not result in interventions to stop the HSB can compound the SSA by letting it persist.

Role of Professionals

To facilitate disclosure professionals need to validate the child and adult survivor's experience and explore what they had to do to survive and how they made sense of what happened to them. This is best achieved if professionals are resourced with a good understanding of the complexity and nuances of SSA through specialist training which enables them to conduct accurate assessments and case formulations, and ensure the use of appropriate and precise language (Yates & Allardyce, 2021). In addition, professionals need to be able to bear witness to the survivor's narrative without judgement, or minimising or catastrophising what has happened to them (McCartan et al., 2021), and be able to feel comfortable listening to and talking about sexuality and child-on-child sexual abuse (Sanderson, 2004, 2013). It is also essential not to dismiss the SSA as less harmful than CSA and to remain empathic and compassionate.

This is particularly important if working with the family and both the sibling who is being harmed and the sibling who has harmed, especially if the sibling who has committed SSA has experienced sexual abuse themselves, and as such has what is called 'dual status' – both a victim of sexual abuse and a child who enacts sexual abuse. To reduce the risk of re-traumatisation, professionals need to be mindful when working with families that this is safe and in the best interest of the child or adult survivor, and assess to what extent the sibling who has harmed is able to accept responsibility for the SSA and apologise for the harm caused, and whether they still exert some power and control over the sibling who is being harmed. Moreover, they need to work within a developmental, relational, trauma-informed practice framework (see Chapter 9) (Sanderson, 2013, 2022; McCartan et al., 2021; Yates & Allardyce, 2021).

Practitioners working with adult survivors of SSA need to be aware that some survivors of SSA will be uncertain as to whether they have been sexually abused or not. Ideally, they need to feel equipped with an understanding of what is developmentally typical sexual exploration and experimentation and what is considered to be atypical sexual behaviour and constitutes HSB and SSA. This will ensure that they do not dismiss or minimise SSA and can enable the survivor to explore how this has impacted them. Alongside this, it is vital that they validate the survivor's experience, even if they did not experience it as abusive at the time.

As many children do not experience SSA as abusive or harmful at the time and do not display overt trauma reactions, they find it hard to recognise their experience as traumatic. Practitioners need to be aware that while not all SSA is experienced as trauma, it nevertheless contains a number of trauma elements which may not manifest until late adolescence or adulthood as delayed trauma. This is also the case for 'dual status' children who have experienced CSA and go on to engage in HSB.

As systematic and repeated exposure to the misuse of power and control, non-consensual sexual experiences and shame underpins complex post-traumatic stress disorder (C-PTSD), practitioners need to adopt a trauma-informed approach when working with adult survivors of SSA. This can be facilitated by a good understanding of trauma and its impact and incorporating the core principles of trauma-informed practice into their therapeutic modality, alongside a phased approach to resource the survivor and pace the therapeutic work (see Chapter 9). Throughout, they need to support this with a relational and strengths-based approach to enable the survivor to heal from SSA and regain relational worth, cultivate relationship skills and a sense of empowerment (see Chapter 10) (Sanderson, 2013, 2022).

The Power Threat Meaning Framework (Johnstone & Boyle, 2018) which focuses on 'what happened' to the survivor, rather than focusing on 'what is wrong with them', will enable practitioners to understand how prolonged exposure to power and control dynamics can impact on the child and the requisite adaptations needed to help them cope with and survive their experiences, and how they extract meaning from what happened to them (see Chapter 9). This will also help them to identify power differentials between siblings and how these were used to coerce or manipulate the sibling who is being harmed, and to assess to what extent the sibling who has harmed still exerts his or her power in adulthood through subterfuge, distortion of reality, provoking divisiveness, scapegoating, or labelling the survivor as being emotionally or mentally unstable.

To ensure that professionals are better equipped to identify, assess, and provide appropriate support and interventions, McCartan et al. (2021) make a number of recommendations including a clear definition of SSA that would allow for separate recording criteria rather than subsuming it under the collective category of SSA as this would enable researchers to gain more accurate prevalence data. This can further facilitate the development of national guidelines and protocols so that professionals are better able to support children and adult survivors who have experienced SSA (McCartan et al., 2021).

Resourcing professionals through specialist training will enable them to develop good practice, when working with children, families, and adult survivors. If this is combined with enhancing awareness of SSA for parents, teachers, children, and the general public through the media, documentaries, TV dramas, podcasts, or sex education, it will uncover the hidden nature of SSA and enable children and adults to give voice to their experiences and gain access to appropriate support (see Chapter 11).

Structure of the Book
Chapter 1 The Nature of Sibling Sexual Abuse
This chapter will examine the nature and dynamics of SSA and how it manifests. It will identify the range of motivations that lead siblings to sexually harm brothers or sisters, including understanding those siblings who have been sexually abused and who go on to abuse their sibling(s). Commonly SSA is seen or experienced as sexual experimentation, and thus normalised. The chapter will explore the role of confusion, sense of complicity, secrecy, and desire to protect the family and the harming sibling which makes it hard for siblings who have been harmed to legitimise the SSA and to disclose. It will explore the myriad barriers

to disclosure such as the desire to preserve the family, or not involve authorities to protect the harming sibling.

Chapter 2 Risk Factors in Sibling Sexual Abuse

This chapter will explore who is most at risk of committing SSA and of being harmed. It will unpack the complex interplay between individual predispositions in the child, neurodivergence, history of previous sexual abuse, trauma, and ACEs, as well as family dynamics, and socio-cultural factors such as race, socio-economic status, poverty, religion, and cultural norms and concomitant expectations. The impact of early exposure to pornography, and how this intersects with regard to problematic sexual behaviour, HSB, or SSA, will be examined alongside how to respond sensitively when supporting parents.

Chapter 3 Typical Sexual Development and Sexual Behaviour in Children and Young People

In order to identify atypical or non-normative psychosexual development and behaviour in children it is necessary to know what is considered to be developmentally typical or normative psychosexual development. This chapter will examine developmentally typical behaviour across three major age groups: 0–4, 5–12, and 13–18. It aims to increase awareness and understanding of normative psychosexual development and behaviour so it can be distinguished from atypical psychosexual development to enable parents and professionals to distinguish between age appropriate consensual sexual activity and HSB in children.

Chapter 4 Atypical Sexual Behaviour in Children and Young People

This chapter will examine the range of HSB and developmentally atypical psychosexual behaviour and how this manifests across three age groups. The chapter will also highlight the range of sexual behaviours in children and young people with learning difficulties, and those who are neurodivergent, and examine to what extent these children are at risk of being sexually abused and displaying problematic or harmful sexual behaviour.

Chapter 5 The Impact of Sibling Sexual Abuse

Chapter 5 will highlight the impact of SSA on both the sibling who has been harmed and the sibling who has caused harm. Although much of

SSA is normalised, and many siblings report little or no harm at the time of the abuse, it will nevertheless have considerable psychobiological impact. Given the proximity of the siblings living under the same roof, and if the SSA is repeated over a prolonged period of time, it can lead to complex trauma (C-PTSD) and developmental trauma disorder which can result in a range of trauma reactions, such as emotional dysregulation, prolonged fear states, dissociation, flashbacks, sleep disturbances, as well as shame, self-blame, and self-harming behaviours. These will be identified and linked to the risk of delayed trauma which can surface later on in life.

Chapter 6 Understanding the Sexually Abused Child

The aim of this chapter is to build on the previous chapter to enable parents and professionals to understand the sexually abused child. It will look at how dissociation manifests in children and how this is often misunderstood or misdiagnosed. It will also explore how dissociation and the SSA impact the developing sense of self, shame, and negative self-perceptions, and how these link to relationship difficulties.

Chapter 7 The Long-Term Effects of Sibling Sexual Abuse on Adult Survivors

This chapter will examine delayed trauma reactions and the risk of post-traumatic stress disorder (PTSD) and C-PTSD in adulthood along with the long-term effects of SSA. It will identify the trauma symptoms associated with SSA such as dissociation, emotional dysregulation, somatisation, compromised physical and mental health, sexual difficulties, as well as the use of substances such as alcohol, drugs, medication, and food to numb overwhelming emotions.

Chapter 8 The Intrapersonal and Relational Effects of Sibling Sexual Abuse in Adult Survivors

This chapter will explore the impact of SSA on the attachment system and relationships, including intimacy and sexuality, and the risk of further re-victimisation. Many survivors of SSA struggle with relationships and, although they yearn for connection, they are also terrified of this, leading to approach–avoid behaviour which can be confusing for them as well as friends and partners. It will also look at how SSA can activate fears of being able to care for and protect their own children when they become parents, and how to navigate family of origin relationships, including with the sibling who harmed them.

Chapter 9 Working with Adult Survivors of Sibling Sexual Abuse: Trauma-Informed Practice

This chapter will consider how to work with adult survivors of SSA within a trauma-informed practice model, which requires an understanding of the Power Threat Meaning Framework (Johnstone & Boyle, 2018) and adoption of a phase-oriented approach to titrate exposure to the SSA experiences. The chapter will focus on how to manage the aftermath of SSA in adulthood, through stabilisation, grounding skills, mindfulness, and breathing in order to master emotional self-regulation in order to enhance distress tolerance so that they are more able to process traumatic experiences and integrate these.

Chapter 10 Working with Adult Survivors of Sibling Sexual Abuse: The Therapeutic Relationship

This chapter will highlight the importance of the power of a healing relationship and its role in building trust, restoring relational worth, and developing relationship skills. It is through the therapeutic relationship that survivors are able to reconnect to self and others, and build healthy relationships. The chapter also explores the myriad challenges of working with survivors of SSA such as vicarious traumatisation and compassion fatigue, and the importance of practitioner self-care to minimise the risk of burnout and secondary traumatic stress.

Chapter 11 The Prevention of Sibling Sexual Abuse

This chapter will explore the range of protective factors that mitigate the risk of being subjected to SSA, as well as reducing the risk of children committing HSB. It will also examine the importance of working with families to improve understanding of HSB, how to set clear boundaries, ensure adequate supervision of children, and how to talk about sex with children and adolescents in an age appropriate way.

Chapter 12 Future Research and Professional Practice

This chapter will identify areas for future research and how to improve professional practice through establishing a clear definition of SSA, developing national guidelines for assessment and treatment intervention, and reporting and recording of SSA. This will increase awareness of SSA among professionals such as social care workers, child protection workers, youth workers, the police, and teachers, as well as mental health professionals, psychologists, and therapists. This in combination with specialist training will ensure that professionals are appropriately resourced to support children, families, and adult survivors of SSA.

Use of Language

Peer-on-peer sexual abuse and sexual violence committed by children on children is termed 'harmful sexual behaviour'. The term HSB is used to distinguish children and young people from adults who commit CSA and ensure that they are not seen as 'mini-adult sex offenders' by acknowledging the child's and young person's developmental status (Hackett et al., 2019; Yates & Allardyce, 2021). It also reflects research findings that indicate that many of those who display HSB do not go on to sexually abuse in adulthood and have very different offending trajectories compared to adult sex offenders (Lussier & Blokland, 2014; McKillop et al., 2015).

In addition, HSB adopts the terms 'child who has been harmed' rather than 'victim/survivor' and 'child who has harmed' rather than 'perpetrator' (McNeish & Scott, 2018) in order to minimise stigmatisation through labelling. In line with this, the language used in this book will be 'the sibling who has been harmed' and 'the sibling who has harmed'. It is important that professionals are able to develop precise language when working with SSA to ensure clarity of understanding among professionals, families, and adult survivors.

Case Illustrations

The case illustrations are all fictionalised examples of what is commonly seen in SSA and how these commonly manifest in clinical practice. Any reader who strongly identifies with any individual case illustration is encouraged to be mindful that these are fictionalised examples rather than any one specific survivor's experience.

Health Warning

As the book contains a number of composite case illustrations commonly seen in SAA, it is important to be aware that some of these may be harrowing to read and may be triggering for some readers. It is important to monitor your reactions to the material and to ensure that you feel safe. If you feel overwhelmed it is essential to pause, take a break, and ground yourself. You can always come back to the book at a later point.

Further Reading

Caffaro, J. (2020). Sibling abuse of other children. In R. Geffner, V. Vieth, V. Vaughan-Eden, A. Rosenbaum, L. Hamberger, & J. White (eds), *Handbook of Interpersonal Violence across the Lifespan*. Springer.

Caffaro, J.V., & Conn-Caffaro, A. (1998). *Sibling abuse trauma: Assessment and intervention strategies for children, families and adults*. Routledge.

Hackett, S. (2001). *Facing the future: A guide for parents of young people who have sexually abused*. Russell House Publishing.

Hackett, S., Balfe, M., Masson, H., & Phillips, J. (2014). Family responses to young people who have sexually abused: Anger, ambivalence and acceptance. *Children & Society*, 28(2), 128–139.

Hackett, S., Branigan, P., & Holmes, D. (2019). *Harmful Sexual Behaviour Framework: An evidence-informed operational framework for children and young people displaying harmful sexual behaviours* (2nd edn). NSPCC.

Hackett, S., Phillips, J., Masson, H., & Balfe, M. (2013). Individual, family and abuse characteristics of 700 British child and adolescent sexual abusers. *Child Abuse Review*, 22(4), 232–245.

McCartan, K., Anning, A., & Qureshi, E. (2021). *The impact of sibling sexual abuse on adults who were harmed as children*. UWE, Bristol Research Report.

Punch, S. (2008). 'You can do nasty things to your brothers and sisters without a reason': Siblings' backstage behaviour. *Children & Society*, 22(5), 333–344.

Sanderson, C. (2004). *The seduction of children: Empowering parents and teachers to protect children from sexual abuse*. Jessica Kingsley Publishers.

Sanderson, C. (2022). *The warrior within: A One in Four handbook to aid recovery for survivors of childhood sexual abuse and violence* (4th edn). One in Four.

White, N., & Hughes, C. (2018). *Why siblings matter: The role of brother and sister relationships in development and well-being*. Routledge.

Yates, P., & Allardyce, S. (2021). *Sibling sexual abuse: Knowledge and practice*. Centre of Expertise on Child Sexual Abuse.

Yates, P., & Allardyce, S. (2022). Abuse at the heart of the family: The challenges and complexities of sibling sexual abuse. In K. Uzieblo, W.J. Smid, & K. McCartan (eds), *Challenges in the Management of People Convicted of a Sexual Offence*. Palgrave Macmillan.

CHAPTER 1

The Nature of Sibling Sexual Abuse

The nature of SSA is complex and consists of the interplay of individual predispositions, family dynamics, and cultural factors. This chapter will examine the nature and dynamics of SSA, how it manifests, who is most at risk of being harmed, and who is at risk of committing SSA. It will also identify the range of motivations that lead siblings to sexually harm their brothers or sisters, including those siblings who have been sexually abused and go on to abuse their sibling(s). The normalisation of SSA, alongside feelings of shame and wanting to protect the sibling who harms and preserve the family, makes it extremely hard for the sibling who has been harmed to disclose. These barriers to disclosure and parental responses to disclosure will be explored alongside potential post-disclosure trauma.

SSA is commonly subsumed under the category of CSA although it is rarely given a separate category when it is reported to statutory agencies, including the police, making it hard to obtain the prevalence of SSA. When cases of SSA are linked to the intergenerational transmission of CSA, and passed down the generations wherein the sibling who has harmed is both a victim of CSA and commits SSA, they are considered to have 'dual status'.

Some researchers consider SSA to be a part of what is considered to be HSB, which is defined as 'sexual behaviours expressed by children and young people under the age of 18 years old that are developmentally inappropriate, may be harmful towards self or others, or be abusive towards another child [or] young person' (Hackett et al., 2019, p. 13) (see Chapter 2).

A number of studies have found that between a quarter and half of HSB involves siblings or close family relatives such as cousins, nephews, and nieces (Shaw et al., 2000; Hardy, 2001; Beckett, 2006; Atwood, 2007; Finkelhor, 2009; Hackett et al., 2019). Furthermore, it is estimated that SSA is three times more common than intergenerational CSA (Wiehe, 1997; Krienert & Walsh, 2011; Stroebel et al., 2013; Caffaro & Conn-Caffaro, 2014) which suggests that SSA could be a hidden and under-reported type of both HSB and CSA.

SSA is poorly understood by parents and professionals, as they often find it hard to understand the nature and dynamics of SSA, its impact and long-term effects. The lack of knowledge of what constitutes typical sexual experimentation between siblings and atypical sexual behaviour (see Chapter 2) leads to a normalisation of sexual activity between siblings, making it harder to legitimise it as abuse, and to lack of reporting. The proximity and opportunity within family settings for systematic SSA, and the likelihood of a greater number of sexual acts, enacted over longer periods of time (O'Brien, 1991; Tidefors et al., 2010; Latzman et al., 2011), as well as secrecy and shame can prevent detection and can lead to developmental trauma disorder (DTD) and C-PTSD, or, in those siblings who do not experience the SSA as abuse or trauma in childhood, delayed trauma as they reach late adolescence or adulthood (see Chapter 3).

In the absence of a clear definition of SSA it is difficult to know precisely what SSA is and the nature of what is understood as 'siblings'. McCartan et al. (2021, p. 6) define SSA as 'any form of sexualized behavior or action, contact and non-contact, between siblings when they were under the age of 18'. As SSA generally refers to children who grow up in the same family whether they are stepchildren, foster children, adopted children, or birth children (Yates & Allardyce, 2021), it is prudent to include not only biological siblings, but also stepsiblings, half siblings, foster siblings, adopted siblings, as well as extended family peers such as cousins.

Research suggests that commonly SSA consists of an older or stronger sibling coercing a younger, smaller, or less strong sibling into sexual activity. While age and physical strength are strong indices, what must not be overlooked is the imbalance of power between siblings in areas such as authority, status, privilege due to being a favoured child, or being in loco parentis. In some cases the SSA is normalised and not perceived as abuse and continues into adulthood (Caffaro, 2017).

The motivation in SSA can also vary enormously from comfort and attachment seeking to rage and jealousy, as can the nature of the sexual activity. It is crucial that parents and practitioners recognise that the experience of SSA is not homogeneous and that to fully comprehend the complex nature of SSA they need to be aware of the unique individual lived experience of each child who has been harmed and the child who is harming.

While the most commonly reported pattern of SSA involves an older brother abusing a younger sister, all combinations of siblings are possible, including same-sex abuse, brother to brother, sister to sister, as well as sisters abusing brothers, younger siblings abusing older siblings, and multiple siblings being abused as intergenerational CSA cascades down from sibling to sibling (Adler & Schutz, 1995; DiGiorgio-Miller, 1998; Carlson et al., 2006; Stroebel et al., 2013; Caffaro & Conn-Caffaro, 2014; O'Keefe et al., 2014). Recent research (McCartan et al., 2021) has highlighted that female SSA may be more pronounced and common than previously identified, with 28% of SSA committed by sisters and not brothers which may indicate that SSA is not necessarily gendered. Historical research indicates that the average age of onset for a sibling to be harmed is nine years (De Jong, 1989; O'Brien, 1991; Laviola, 1992) and the peak age is thought to be between 12 and 14 years old (Finkelhor, 2009). This data may no longer be representative of the current landscape of SSA and requires more current research.

With regard to the impact of SSA, there is currently insufficient evidence with regard to the degree of harm caused by each of the different gender combinations, or how the impact of SSA compares to intergenerational CSA, although some researchers argue that SSA has the potential to be every bit as harmful as sexual abuse by parents (Yates, 2017; Yates & Allardyce, 2021).

The Dynamics of Sibling Sexual Abuse

SSA is part of a spectrum of sibling interactions and relationships which can include emotional, physical, and sexual abuse. While many sibling relationships are positive and growth promoting, and non-abusive (Yates & Allardyce, 2021), some are abusive and can cause significant harm. The impact of sibling relationships has been largely under-researched which has led to a poor understanding of the spectrum of sibling relationships especially with regard to abusive behaviour. This is exacerbated by lack of understanding what constitutes abusive behaviour, with some families actively encouraging teasing which can easily tip over into bullying, while play fighting can turn into physical abuse, and sexual curiosity can transmute into SSA.

Families may not be aware of what is happening due to the normalisation of sexual experimentation or a sense of complicity which silences the sibling who is being harmed, preventing disclosure and reporting. In addition, some siblings who commit SSA groom both the sibling who is being harmed as well as other family members, including parent(s), in order to remain undetected.

Normalisation of Sexual Activity between Siblings

Children are naturally curious about the world, their body, and the bodies of others. As part of their development of knowledge about themselves they explore their own bodies and seek to compare their body to others. This leads to normative sexual exploration and experimentation as part of their psychosexual development. Such normative exploration and sexual play is consensual, mutual, and fun with much giggling and hilarity. This is significantly different to HSB and SSB. Many parents and professionals are not able to distinguish between typical sexual exploration and atypical sexual behaviour. As a result sexual activity between siblings is often normalised, leaving the child and later survivor in a state of confusion and doubt about what happened to them. Such normalisation can result in a lack of recognition of abuse in childhood, and lead to delayed trauma in adulthood.

> ### Conrad
> Conrad was sexually abused by his brother between the ages of five and eight, who repeatedly told him that this was normal and not abusive. It was not until Conrad started dating when he was 18 and experienced sexual difficulties, confusion, and self-loathing that he tried to make sense of his experiences. Initially he was unable to link his revulsion around sex to what happened to him, until he started to explore this in therapy.

In order to prevent the normalisation of SSA it is essential to distinguish between consensual sexual experimentation and harmful sexual behaviour, and to understand the difference between what is generally considered to be typical and atypical psychosexual development in children and young people (see Chapters 3 and 4). This allows for greater awareness of what is age appropriate consensual sexual curiosity and experimentation, and what is atypical sexual behaviour which is non-consensual and sexually harmful.

SSA, even when normalised, is shrouded in secrecy and silence, making it hard to disclose it for fear of the consequences. The need to keep the secret and remain silent means there is no opportunity to reality check whether such sexual activity is normal, leaving the sibling being harmed confused and subject to overwhelming feelings, with no access to support or comfort. The sense of *knowing that something is wrong* and the need *not to know* this for fear of the consequences means that the child has to split off what is happening to them so they can preserve their belief that the sibling who is harming them is good and does not mean to harm them. In addition, the fear of the secret being exposed means they have to lead a double life wherein they become invisible to avoid the abuse, or develop a false self to hide the shame and wounded inner self. This can lead to an avoidance of making friends or developing close relationships in case the secret is exposed, leading to isolation and loneliness as they become locked into a psychological prison.

The Grooming Process

As in CSA, the grooming process is designed to entice the sibling into a 'special relationship' while at the same time undermining any attachment to primary caregivers or other siblings. As the grooming is often so subtle and gradual, the sibling who is being harmed perceives this as a normal part of a special relationship and is unable to question it. As the sexual contact escalates and the sibling who is being harmed has no other source of secure attachment, he or she has no choice but to submit. The special relationship is cemented by paying the sibling who is being harmed extra attention, or allowing them to play with them or join in their games. These games are often fun and the sibling who is being harmed enjoys being included by the sibling who has harmed and relishes spending time with them, and being liked and accepted, rather than being batted away as a nuisance. While initially these games do not contain sexual elements, they tend to become more sexualised over time. Commonly such games involve some initiation ritual or forfeits such as removing clothes or having to do something that is inappropriate.

Lara

Lara was excited that her older brothers allowed her to join in their games as normally they excluded her and shut her out of their room. As she adored her brothers and wanted to be close to them she was willing to do whatever was asked of her. While she didn't really understand the rules of the games and often lost, she willingly performed whatever forfeits her brothers requested. Initially this entailed removing layers of clothing, and once naked, touching herself sexually which one of her brothers filmed. Eventually she was required to sexually touch one of her brothers and engage in sexual intercourse while the other brother filmed this.

To minimise the risk of exposure, some siblings who have harmed also go on to groom other family members by inserting doubt in the mind of the sibling who is being harmed about how much they are really cared for by the parent(s) or other siblings while simultaneously sowing seeds of doubt in the parent's mind about how much the sibling who is being harmed can be trusted to be truthful. As a result both the sibling who is being harmed and the non-abusing parent(s) are groomed to not trust each other, which reduces the risk of disclosure and the likelihood that the sibling who is being harmed will be believed. In driving a wedge between the sibling who is being harmed and the family, the sibling who has harmed is able to 'divide and rule' and prevent the child from disclosing the abuse. As the bond between the sibling who is being harmed and other family members dissolves, the bond between the sibling who is being harmed and sibling who has harmed is strengthened, creating a trauma bond which makes the child more dependent on the sibling who has harmed.

A trauma bond is most likely to occur when there is an imbalance of power, in which one person has control and authority over another, and when caring and affectionate behaviour alternates with physical, emotional, or sexual abuse. As the sibling who is being harmed becomes more dependent on the sibling who has harmed he or she is compelled to seal off any negative beliefs about the harming sibling through 'thought blindness' in which they disavow the abuse components in order to focus on the positive and caring aspects of the sibling who has harmed, so as to humanise rather than demonise them. In focusing on the loving aspects of the abuser the sibling who is being harmed sees the sibling who has harmed as 'good' and themselves as 'bad'. As the dependency on the sibling who has harmed increases the trauma bond becomes the 'superglue that bonds' the relationship, which is so strong that anything that may threaten that bond will be resisted (Sanderson, 2013, 2022), including any potential exposure or disclosure of the SSA.

Dynamics in Feeling Complicit

During the process of grooming abuse masquerades as love and affection which distorts the reality of the sibling who is being harmed, as it normalises sexual activity between siblings and changes the sense of self of the sibling who is being harmed and their ability to trust and relate to others (see Chapter 6). It also makes the sibling who is being harmed feel complicit in the SSA which reduces the risk of disclosure. Feeling complicit prevents the sibling who is being harmed from legitimising their abuse and confines them to suffering in silence, with no support either from their family or professionals. In not being able to verbalise what is happening to them they find it harder to make sense of their experiences which in turn prevents them from processing their experiences.

The sibling who is being harmed can feel complicit in wanting to spend time with the sibling who has harmed, and seeking them out to play with them. The need to be liked and approved of can lead to appeasement behaviour and compliance which the sibling who is being harmed misconstrues as wanting and accepting the SSA. This complicity is compounded if they have enjoyed aspects of the sexual activity or became aroused. If the sibling who is being harmed experienced sexual pleasure, had an erection, became lubricated, or had an orgasm they will interpret this as having wanted the sexual encounter. It is crucial that siblings who are being harmed are provided with psychoeducation that any arousal and sexual responses are normal psychobiological responses to being touched in certain parts of the body that are elicited outside of voluntary control and do not indicate sexual desire (Sanderson, 2004, 2013, 2022).

Range of Sexual Behaviours in Sibling Sexual Abuse

The range of sexual behaviours associated with SSA includes both non-contact and contact behaviours. Some siblings are enticed into looking at sexually explicit material and images, including pornography, which can have a dis-inhibitory effect in normalising sexual contact between children, or children and adults. The sibling who has harmed may also engage in voyeurism or exhibitionism including masturbating in front of the sibling who is being harmed, or encouraging them to masturbate. Non-contact behaviour can also consist of filming the sibling who is being harmed while naked, or touching themselves, or masturbating and posting it online on social media. Such images can also be used to advertise the sexual availability of the sibling who is being harmed for further sexual exploitation.

Some SSA can begin with sexual experimentation and sexual play which can over time escalate into HSB (Canavan et al., 1992; Carlson et al., 2006). Sexual exploratory play commonly consists of looking, touching, rubbing, stroking, or kissing the genital area, either directly or through clothing, which invariably feels nice and pleasurable. Conversely, some SSA occurs without any sexual play and consists of non-consensual sexual activity driven by power and control such as masturbation, mutual masturbation, oral genital contact, simulated or attempted vaginal or anal penetration, or vaginal or anal penetration (see Chapter 4).

The duration of the SSA can also vary enormously, with some occurring only once, or intermittently or daily. Some SSA can start as developmentally normative sexual play within an appropriate developmental stage which the sibling who has harmed outgrows as they mature, while for others it continues over many years, straddling a number of developmental stages, gradually escalating in terms of frequency and severity of HSB as the sibling who has harmed enters puberty.

Spectrum of Motivation in Sibling Sexual Interactions

Siblings who commit SSA are not homogeneous and will vary considerably in their motivation to engage in HSB (see Box 1.1). Some siblings may just be curious and engage in sexual exploration and sexual play. While this is considered to be typical sexual behaviour in children under the age of five, this may persist beyond certain developmental stages either because the siblings have become frozen in a particular stage, or because the behaviour has become conditioned and normalised.

Children who live in adverse or chaotic family environments may huddle together to soothe and comfort each other, which can become sexualised.

Carol

Carol's parents struggled with alcohol and drug addiction and would invariably be intoxicated throughout the day and evening while partying with other addicts. Carol and her siblings were frequently left to their own devices, with Carol acting as a surrogate mother. After feeding and bathing her siblings in the evening, they would all curl up together in bed. As the siblings often found it hard to settle, Carol would stroke their genitals to soothe them until they fell asleep. Over time this escalated to the siblings stimulating her and increasingly sexualised behaviour.

Box 1.1 Spectrum of motivation in sibling sexual abuse

- Curiosity, sexual experimentation and sexual play
- Comfort – cuddling, touching, stroking, licking
- Sexual gratification – masturbation, mutual masturbation
- Corruption of innocence – in being abused, or forcing the sibling who is being harmed to perform sexual acts on them
- Sense of entitlement and sense they can do no wrong
- Scapegoating the already scapegoated sibling
- Conditioning of sexual arousal to aggression
- Envy, anger, and rage – retaliation, symbolic way of punishing and annihilating sibling
- Dual status – re-enactment of own sexual abuse, mastery, 'triumph over trauma', defence against shame
- Assertion of power and control – domination, display of power and strength to assuage own powerlessness
- Playing victim – sometimes used to elicit empathy which is then manipulated and exploited
- Distributing sexual images due to being coerced by peers, or to gain approval of peers, or for further sexual exploitation

Some siblings are motivated by envy, anger, and rage.

Chantelle

Eleven-year-old Chantelle looked forward to finally meeting her older brother who had been raised outside the family. She was excited to meet him and was looking forward to spending time with him as she felt he was lonely not having been part of the family. While initially her brother played fun games with her, they became increasingly sexualised, culminating in violent rape. Chantelle wanted to protect her brother as she didn't want him to be sent away and banished from the family again. She believed she had no choice but to endure this until she was old enough to leave home. This need to protect the sibling, especially if they have been rejected or scapegoated, is not uncommon, especially if the sibling who has harmed manipulates this by adopting a victim role to elicit empathy and compassion.

Siblings can also take sexual advantage of another sibling purely because they can, or because the sibling who is being harmed is defined as the family scapegoat, or because the sibling who has harmed is the favoured child who can do no wrong in their parents' view, leading to a sense of entitlement to do as they please without fear of being held accountable.

Sonia

Sonia was sexually abused by her younger brother. Despite being younger, her brother was considerably bigger and stronger than Sonia, and the favoured child who could do no wrong. Her brother had watched porn from a young age and insisted that she should imitate some of the sexual acts she had seen with him. Given his status in the family, Sonia felt she could not tell her parents as she feared she would be made to feel responsible, given that she was older than her brother and should have stopped him. Sonia felt she had no choice but to submit, especially when he started to threaten her physically. Sonia blamed herself as she entered her late teens as she believed that because she did not stop the abuse she was to blame for the SSA.

Some siblings are envious of younger siblings' innocence and want to destroy this either through SSA or by forcing the sibling who is being harmed to either procure other children for them, or coercing him or her to perform sexual acts on other children. This is a powerful strategy on the part of the sibling who has harmed as it places the sibling who is being harmed into the position of committing HSB.

Connor

Connor's older brother repeatedly raped him and also coerced him to commit harmful sexual acts on his peers. Connor's shame and guilt was such that he could not see his brother as abusive or acknowledge the harm done to him, as he believed himself to be no better than his brother in sexually harming other children. This made it very difficult to separate out the harm done to him and the sexual harm he committed on others. The sense of shame was so crippling he was unable to legitimise the SSA he experienced, or access any self-compassion.

Siblings who seek the approval of peers may engage in SSA by filming their siblings engaging in sexual acts and posting these on social media.

Some SSA occurs as a result of the intergenerational transmission of CSA which can cascade through the family and result in SSA, as seen in Selina's family.

Selina

Selina along with her siblings had all been sexually abused by their father, causing significant harm to all the siblings, although all of them minimised its impact. Selina's CSA was further compounded by an older sibling, who also sexually harmed her, leaving her feeling even more betrayed and abandoned.

Selina's sister is an apt example of what is known as 'dual status' siblings who have experienced sexual abuse either by an adult or another sibling, and subsequently go on to sexually abuse a younger sibling or other children. Thus, they are both a victim of sexual abuse and someone who has engaged in HSB. This can create added complexity in terms of empathy and compassion for having experienced sexual abuse while also promoting the need to be held accountable and take responsibility for the HSB committed, and engaging in treatment.

Professionals need to be mindful that although some siblings with a history of sexual abuse may display HSB because of previous abuse (Stathopoulos, 2012), this does not mean that previous sexual abuse causes or predicts future HSB (Stripe & Stermac, 2003). The belief that people who experience CSA go on to sexually abuse is erroneous as the majority of people who have been sexually abused do not go on to sexually abuse. While it is important to acknowledge that some children who experience sexual harm may also engage in HSB or SSA, this is not a given and professionals should not collude with this myth by assuming that there is an inevitable link between the two (Glaser, 1991; Wiehe, 1998; Caspi, 2011; McCartan et al., 2021; Yates & Allardyce, 2021). It is worth noting that while not all siblings who engage in SSA have been sexually abused they may however have experienced relational trauma, broken attachments, physical or emotional abuse, or some other type of trauma, and that the SSA is a way of reclaiming power and control and to gain mastery over what happened to them which might enable them to triumph over trauma.

Given the spectrum of motivations seen in SSA, parents and professionals need to avoid making simplistic assumptions and delve a little deeper into the complex nature and motivations associated with SSA to fully understand both the sibling who is being harmed and the sibling who has harmed. It also helpful to be aware of the risk factors in SSA which will be examined in the next chapter.

Further Reading

Caffaro, J. (2020). Sibling abuse of other children. In R. Geffner, V. Vieth, V. Vaughan-Eden, A. Rosenbaum, L. Hamberger, & J. White (eds), *Handbook of Interpersonal Violence across the Lifespan*. Springer.

Caffaro, J.V., & Conn-Caffaro, A. (1998). *Sibling abuse trauma: Assessment and intervention strategies for children, families and adults*. Routledge.

Hackett, S. (2001). *Facing the future: A guide for parents of young people who have sexually abused*. Russell House Publishing.

Hackett, S., Balfe, M., Masson, H., & Phillips, J. (2014). Family responses to young people who have sexually abused: Anger, ambivalence and acceptance. *Children & Society*, 28(2), 128–139.

Hackett, S., Branigan, P., & Holmes, D. (2019). *Harmful Sexual Behaviour Framework: An evidence-informed operational framework for children and young people displaying harmful sexual behaviours* (2nd edn). NSPCC.

Hackett, S., Phillips, J., Masson, H., & Balfe, M. (2013). Individual, family and abuse characteristics of 700 British child and adolescent sexual abusers. *Child Abuse Review*, 22(4), 232–245.

McCartan, K., Anning, A., & Qureshi, E. (2021). *The impact of sibling sexual abuse on adults who were harmed as children*. UWE, Bristol Research Report.

Sanderson, C. (2006). *Counselling adult survivors of child sexual abuse* (3rd edn). Jessica Kingsley Publishers.

Sanderson, C. (2013). *Counselling skills for working with trauma*. Jessica Kingsley Publishers.

Sanderson, C. (2015). *Counselling skills for working with shame*. Jessica Kingsley Publishers.

Sanderson, C. (2022). *The warrior within: A One in Four handbook to aid recovery for survivors of childhood sexual abuse and violence* (4th edn). One in Four.

Yates, P. (2017). Sibling sexual abuse: Why don't we talk about it? *Journal of Clinical Nursing*, 26(15–16), 2482–2494.

Yates, P., & Allardyce, S. (2021). *Sibling sexual abuse: Knowledge and practice*. Centre of Expertise on Child Sexual Abuse.

Yates, P., & Allardyce, S. (2022). Abuse at the heart of the family: The challenges and complexities of sibling sexual abuse. In K. Uzieblo, W.J. Smid, & K. McCartan (eds), *Challenges in the Management of People Convicted of a Sexual Offence*. Palgrave Macmillan.

CHAPTER 2

Risk Factors in Sibling Sexual Abuse

Some researchers consider SSA to be a part of what is considered to be HSB which is defined as 'sexual behaviours expressed by children and young people under the age of 18 years old that are developmentally inappropriate, may be harmful towards self or others, or be abusive towards another child [or] young person' (Hackett et al., 2019, p. 13). This definition encompasses both on and offline behaviour such as technology-assisted HSB (TA-HSB) as well as contact sexual behaviours and sexual exploitation (Hollis & Belton, 2017).

TA-HSB is further defined as 'sexualised behaviour which children or young people engage in using the internet or technology such as mobile phones' and includes viewing pornography (including extreme pornography or viewing indecent images of children) (NSPCC, 2021, p. 5). Both these definitions emphasise the harm to the child who is harming as well as the child who has been harmed.

While currently under-researched, TA-HSB can lead to a range of developmentally inappropriate sexual behaviours, from engaging in sexual discussions or acts, image-creating, sharing or communication which is inappropriate and/or harmful due to age or stage of development, using or exposing other, younger children to these, through to sexual harassment, grooming, and HSB. In addition, the long-term effect of exposure to pornography can affect the ability to build healthy sexual relationships in adulthood.

The term HSB is used to distinguish children and young people from adults who commit CSA to ensure that they are not seen as 'mini-adult sex offenders' by acknowledging the child's and young person's developmental status. It also reflects research findings that indicate that many of those who display HSB do not go on to sexually abuse in adulthood and have very different offending trajectories compared to adult sex offenders (Lussier & Blokland, 2014; McKillop et al., 2015). In addition, HSB adopts the terms 'child who has been harmed' rather than 'victim/survivor' and 'child who has harmed' rather than 'perpetrator' (McNeish & Scott, 2018) in order to minimise stigmatisation through labelling.

The Scale of Harmful Sexual Behaviour

To date, there are no officially published statistics on the prevalence of HSB, its causes or the characteristics of young people who display this behaviour. Current data estimates that between one-fifth and three-quarters of CSA is committed by children and young people under the age of 18 (Erooga & Masson, 2006; Vizard et al., 2007; Hackett et al., 2014), which is often hidden due to fear of disclosure and shame.

While HSB is most commonly associated with adolescent boys (Vizard et al., 2007; Hackett et al., 2013), girls and younger children also exhibit HSB, along with children with neuroatypical presentations, with over a third of children who are referred with HSB having learning difficulties (Hackett et al., 2013). According to Allardyce and Yates (2018), girls who display HSB are often identified at a younger age, are more likely to have a history of trauma and CSA, and while more likely to harm younger children they tend to use penetration less compared to boys.

Who Is at Risk of Exhibiting Harmful Sexual Behaviour?

Research has identified a number of factors that increase the risk of HSB, most notably a history of severe trauma (Vizard et al., 2007; Hackett et al., 2013), a history of ACEs, including physical and sexual abuse, neglect, and domestic abuse (Tougas et al., 2016), alongside disrupted attachments (Barra et al., 2018).

While some children and young people may be both a 'child who has been harmed' and a 'child who is harming', it is imperative that professionals acknowledge that not all children who display HSB have been sexually abused, nor do they become sexual offenders in adulthood (Hackett et al., 2019). Research has shown that the most strongly associated risk factors are a history of trauma and disrupted attachments, rather than CSA specifically. It is critical that forensic and child protection services take this into consideration when assessing the risk of HSB in the future and recommending effective interventions. In addition, neurodivergent children are also more at risk of committing HSB or SSA (see Chapter 4).

A further risk of HSB is the use of pornography and how this links to 'acting out' or 'mimicking' what has been viewed (Mead & Sharpe, 2017). Cundy (2015) found that 53% of 11–16-year-olds viewed sexually explicit material online, while Sabina et al. (2008) found that 17.9% of males and 10.2% of females under the age of 18 viewed pornography depicting rape or sexual violence, and 15.1% of males and 8.9% of females reported viewing child abuse images. Although to date, there is insufficient empirical data to assess the relative contribution of TA-HSB to HSB, research is needed to identify links between online TA-HSB and offline HSB.

Harmful sexual behaviour occurs on a continuum of sexual behaviours, ranging from normative sexual behaviour, to inappropriate or problematic sexual behaviour, through to abusive and violent sexual abuse (Hackett, 2010, see Table 2.1). Characteristics associated with HSB include preoccupation with sexual expression and compulsive sexual activity, exhibitionism, and voyeurism, with the child not easily distracted from the sexual activity. It is also non-consensual and can include elements of coercion, deception, enticement, intimidation, threat, as well as aggression, physical force, or violence.

When categorising the nature of the HSB, it is crucial to take into account developmental factors such as age, intellectual or emotional maturity, power imbalances, assigned status, and gender (Hackett, 2010), and to have awareness that some behaviours that are considered typical in one developmental stage may be a cause of concern at a different developmental stage (Friedrich et al., 1998; Ryan, 2000), as well as having a knowledge of developmental factors in neurodivergent children. Practitioners also need to take cultural factors and how these intersect into consideration.

Young children who display HSB are generally more likely to display 'inappropriate' or 'problematic' HSB, whereas adolescents are more likely to display 'abusive' or 'violent' which is often predicated on the use of power, lack of consent, and the use of force, coercion, and threats, as well as secrecy, degradation, and the use of grooming and dis-inhibitors such as drugs or alcohol (McNeish & Scott, 2018; Yates & Allardyce, 2021). Bentovim et al. (2009) found that children who displayed HSB below age 11 were not predominantly sexually motivated, and more likely to be fuelled by a need for power and control to counteract their sense of powerlessness, humiliation, and own abuse histories. This can subsequently become increasingly sexualised, especially as they go into puberty. Children over the age of 11 tend to be much more sexually motivated especially when they have entered puberty as this fuses with compensatory strategies to assert themselves and overcome the sense of powerlessness.

Research has traditionally viewed SSA as a gendered form of abuse with the most commonly reported being brother to sister; it is also seen in brother to brother, sister to sister, and sister to brother, albeit less often reported. This may be due to gendered differences with regard to reporting and help seeking, as well as societal attitudes towards females and the belief they are less likely to sexually abuse. McCartan et al.'s (2021) study found that a large proportion of SSA was committed by females, suggesting SSA is not inherently linked to gender.

Sibling sexual abuse can occur in any family and be experienced and committed by both genders. The vulnerability to SSA may be elevated if there is a history of CSA in the family which has been normalised for both adults and children. While it is not a given that this will result in HSB to others, there are examples where SSA cascades throughout the family in which siblings irrespective of gender are at risk. This is seen in families where a parent or parents sexually abuse one or several children, some of whom then go on to sexually abuse their younger siblings.

Claudia

Claudia and several of her siblings were sexually abused by Claudia's father. The eldest sibling went on to abuse the younger siblings, who in turn went on to abuse the youngest siblings. As each of the siblings experienced abuse, they all normalised the sexual behaviour and never discussed what happened to them. Despite the normalisation, each sibling lived in shame and silence, believing that they needed to keep the secret from each other, until Claudia broke the silence. This caused huge ruptures in the family with some of the siblings wishing to repair and heal together and others wishing to continue to deny the abuse experiences, leading to seismic fractures in the family, and the scapegoating of Claudia for revealing the secret.

Table 2.1 Continuum of children and young people's sexual behaviour (Hackett, 2010)

Normal	Inappropriate	Problematic	Abusive	Violent
Developmentally expected	Single instances of inappropriate sexual behaviour	Problematic and concerning behaviours	Victimising intent or outcome	Physically violent sexual abuse
Socially acceptable	Socially acceptable behaviour within peer group	Developmentally unusual and socially unexpected	Includes misuse of power	Highly intrusive
Consensual, mutual, reciprocal			Coercion and force to ensure victim compliance	Instrumental violence which is physiologically and/or sexually arousing to the perpetrator
Shared decision making	Context for behaviour may be inappropriate	No overt elements of victimisation	Intrusive	Sadism
	Generally consensual and reciprocal	Consent issues may be unclear	Informed consent lacking or not able to be freely given by victim	
		May lack reciprocity or equal power		
		May include levels of compulsivity	May include elements of expressive violence	

Predisposing Factors to Commit Sibling Sexual Abuse

The risk of committing SSA is shaped by multiple factors on multiple levels and is dependent on the interplay between individual predispositions, exposure to trauma, as well as family dynamics, ecological factors, and wider societal and cultural influences (Caffaro, 2020). What is not clear is the relative contribution of each of the factors, and it is imperative that professionals do not ascribe responsibility to any one particular factor to the exclusion of others. The need is to be aware of the interplay between individual and systemic factors in each case rather than shame or blame the child, the family, or the society or culture.

Individual factors that are associated with risk of committing SSA include the age and gender of the sibling who is being harmed and the age of the sibling who has harmed, as well as the nature of the sibling relationship. Additional factors include physical size and strength differentials as well as intelligence, cognitive capacity, and developmental sophistication. The imbalance of power, status, and authority is a crucial factor in the misuse of power (Caffaro, 2017) and gaining dominance over the sibling who is being harmed, as it enables the sibling who has harmed to attain compliance and submission (Cyr et al., 2002; Courtois & Ford, 2012; Stroebel et al., 2013; Caffaro & Conn-Caffaro, 2014).

Physical, sexual, or relational trauma, severe neglect, and a history of broken or disrupted attachments are all potential risk factors for SSA. The concomitant unmet emotional or physical needs can lead siblings to attach to each other, and to huddle together for comfort which can transmute into sexual activities. Children who have experienced myriad broken attachments and feel neglected or abandoned may feel envy or jealousy towards siblings, leading to resentment, anger, and rage, which they try to expunge by humiliating or sexually harming others. Children who experience role confusion in having to act as surrogate or substitute parents, and as such are having to carry too much responsibility, may feel resentful as they are expected to behave like pseudo-adults to the detriment of being free to be a child. Such resentment can lead to wanting to punish or corrupt younger siblings and strip them of their innocence.

Direct exposure to and witnessing of adult sexual behaviour in the home or through pornography, social media, films, and music can lead to premature sexualisation and excitation. This can be arousing and lead to a desire to mimic such sexual behaviour with someone who is easily coerced and compliant such as a younger sibling. This is often the case in neurodivergent children, or those with learning difficulties or mental and physical challenges.

Family Factors Associated with Committing Sibling Sexual Abuse

Individual factors are further influenced and shaped by family dynamics. While there is evidence that family dysfunction can have a significant impact on the risk of SSA, this is correlational rather than causal as they do not fully account for all SSA. While SSA is correlated with dysfunctional families, it does not occur in all dysfunctional families (Caffaro, 2017). Conversely SSA also occurs in functional families where parents are physically and emotionally present. It can also occur in families where a parent or caregiver has experienced sexual abuse in childhood, which can evoke powerful and overwhelming emotional reactions.

Parents who are survivors of CSA may be hyper-aware of sexualised behaviour between siblings and have strong reactions to any kind of sexual expression, even if developmentally appropriate, and view this as intrinsically atypical or abusive. Conversely, some may be confused about appropriate sexual boundaries between siblings, and be uncertain how to manage these, or do not acknowledge the seriousness of SSA, thereby denying or minimising it, leaving both siblings unsupported (Yates & Allardyce, 2021). Furthermore Yates and Allardyce (2021) note that some parents may themselves have engaged in HSB or SSA in childhood and thus normalise such behaviour.

Some families may not be aware of SSA while others may know but not realise that it is SSA as they may believe it to be normal sexual experimentation rather than SSA, or have no idea how to manage it or where to go for help. Some parents may know but choose not to act or minimise the SSA as they feel ashamed, and fear the consequences of reporting it. Like the sibling who is being harmed, many parents fear what would happen to the sibling who has harmed and wish to protect him or her, are unsure how to manage split loyalties, and worry that the family will disintegrate. In such cases it is sometimes safer to preserve the 'functional dysfunctionality' of the family systems (McCartan et al., 2021).

Common family dynamics associated with SSA are chaotic and disengaged families, characterised by emotionally absent and detached parenting and lack of parental supervision and intervention (see Table 2.2). Environmental factors such as siblings sharing bedrooms and having large amounts of unstructured and unsupervised time may also contribute to the risk of SSA (Griffee et al., 2016). The reasons that parents may not be emotionally or physically present for considerable periods of time can vary enormously from financial reasons – needing to work long hours or several jobs – to mental health difficulties or alcohol or drug dependency. Whatever the reason, the lack of physical and emotional availability of parents reduces parental supervision, as well as appropriate interventions. It can also lead to confused and confusing parental roles with one sibling being left in charge to act in loco parentis, which creates a power imbalance between siblings that can be misused.

This was Yolande's experience, whose mother worked at night leaving her older sister, Cynthia, in charge of the other siblings.

Yolande

Yolande's sister Cynthia, as the first born, was the favoured child and was given the power to manage and control her younger siblings. Whenever her mother was out at work Cynthia would physically discipline the younger siblings and, once they were in bed, would threaten Yolande with physical punishment unless she submitted to performing sexual acts. Yolande was too terrified to tell her mother about the physical discipline of the younger siblings or the SSA as she feared she would not be believed given the elevated status accorded to her sister.

Detached, indifferent, and inconsistent parenting invariably leads to insecure or broken attachments which increases the need to bond with available siblings to find some sort of comfort and safety, which creates opportunities for the development of a trauma bond and SSA. Absent parenting can also lead to lack of appropriate or unclear boundaries (Canavan et al., 1992; Adler & Schutz, 1995; Tidefors et al., 2010; Yates et al., 2012; Caffaro, 2014; Caffaro, 2017) with regard to physical and tactile behaviour, personal space, and sexual boundaries such as witnessing sexual activity between parents (e.g. Loredo, 1982; Smith & Israel, 1987; Adler & Schutz, 1995; Worling, 1995; Hardy, 2001; Latzman et al., 2011). In conclusion, absent or detached parenting increases the opportunity for abuse and makes it harder to disclose.

Other family dynamics include exposure to coercive controlling behaviour, or aggressive and violent behaviour as in physical or domestic abuse, which normalises violence which can become eroticised. This is often accompanied by problematic and antisocial attitudes in the household such as patriarchal and misogynistic views alongside a lack of respect, lack of voice, and enforced compliance. The lack of voice prevents any open communication between adults and children which leads to the normalisation of silence and secrecy.

Exposure to and experience of other forms of trauma such as ACEs will have a significant impact on physical and mental health. These include physical, sexual, or emotional abuse, emotional and physical neglect, domestic abuse, parental substance abuse, parental mental health problems, and absence of one parent either through separation or incarceration. Any one of these will impact on the family system, and in the case of four or more ACEs can lead to impaired mental and physical health, and give rise to further dysfunction in the family, including a cycle of abuse and SSA in which children imitate abusive behaviours they have witnessed and normalise these. Thus, they may copy physical aggression, or inappropriate sexual behaviour, or misuse power through the use of language, defining other siblings, and the use of coercion or threat to obtain compliance (McCartan et al., 2021).

Table 2.2 Summary of risk factors associated with SSA

Individual	**Family**	**Socio-cultural**
Premature sexualisation – digitisation of sex, social media, pornography Exposure to violence – eroticised rage, humiliation, and shame Impaired attachment Lack of appropriate sexual information Social isolation, rejection, and loneliness Lack of social skills, poor peer relationships, poor anger management skills Neurodivergent or learning disability (40%) Previous sexual victimisation	Emotionally absent parenting Chaotic and disengaged families Relational trauma – impaired or broken attachments Lack of parental supervision ACEs Family sexualised environment Power imbalance between siblings Rigid gender roles Lack of open communication Coercive and controlling behaviour Antisocial attitudes in the household Poor parenting and social skills Lack of appropriate boundaries Aggressive and violent behaviour Poor mental health and/or addictions Parental history of CSA or SSA	Cultural norms and expectations Race Religion Poverty Impoverished social environments Lack of community Racism and discrimination Marginalisation and stigmatisation Sexualisation of children Exposure to pornography and age inappropriate sexual content TA-HSB

Socio-Cultural Factors

There are a number of complex socio-cultural and psychosocial factors such as culture, discrimination, and exposure to pornography which can influence the experiences of the sibling who has harmed and render him or her vulnerable to committing SSA (Yates & Allardyce, 2022). Cultural factors shape family identities and family systems, as well as the individuals in them. When assessing and working with SSA, professionals need to consider race, ethnicity, cultural norms and expectations, socio-economic, educational, and religious factors along with discrimination and marginalisation and how these intersect and impact on family identities (Caffaro, 2020). In addition, they need to be aware of cultural attitudes and beliefs around children and sexuality, the sexualisation of children and restrictions on sexual play, sexual expression, and masturbation (Shah, 2017; McCartan et al., 2021; Yates & Allardyce, 2021). This is essential in order to provide effective family interventions that take into account cultural norms and expectations and the role of honour, as well as incorporating the strengths and resources different cultures provide to avoid adopting a one-size-fits-all approach.

The exposure to pornography and age inappropriate sexual content is also a contributing factor for HSB and SSA and may account for an increase in peer-on-peer and sibling sexual abuse. The easy access of pornography on mobile phones and other devices, especially by increasingly younger children, can lead to premature sexualisation and excitation (Sanderson, 2004) and promote the imitation of sexual acts viewed, including the use of aggression and violence. While some children and young people may enact these with peers, some may entice younger siblings as these may be easier to access and manipulate.

Children who are neurodivergent, or have learning difficulties or face mental and physical challenges, are more vulnerable to being sexually abused or sexually exploited by adults, children, and siblings. Research has shown that children with disabilities are more likely to be sexually abused than neurotypical children (Kelly, 1992; Department of Health, 2000; NSPCC, 2003) with Wissink et al. (2015) finding a three- to four-fold greater likelihood of CSA. Such children are often targeted as they are thought to be less likely to comprehend what is happening to them and less able to verbalise or disclose their experiences. In addition, they may also be less likely to be believed if a disclosure is made, or put on the child protection register.

Very young, pre-verbal children are also at an increased risk of SSA as they do not have the language to communicate what is happening to them, or the cognitive capacity to understand what is happening, which reduces the chance of detection of SSA. A further at-risk group is looked-after children who may be at risk of being sexually abused either in children's homes or by foster siblings in foster homes or when adopted, especially if they have a history of CSA in their family of origin, or have been sexually abused while in care by either adult staff or peers.

In order to be able to assess SSA and distinguish between developmentally appropriate and inappropriate sexual behaviour in children, parents and professionals need to be able to distinguish between normative, consensual sexual play and experimentation in children, and HSB. The following two chapters will explore developmentally typical sexual behaviour, followed by developmentally atypical sexual behaviour.

Further Reading

Caffaro, J. (2020). Sibling abuse of other children. In R. Geffner, V. Vieth, V. Vaughan-Eden, A. Rosenbaum, L. Hamberger, & J. White (eds), *Handbook of Interpersonal Violence across the Lifespan*. Springer.

Caffaro, J.V., & Conn-Caffaro, A. (1998). *Sibling abuse trauma: Assessment and intervention strategies for children, families and adults*. Routledge.

Hackett, S. (2001). *Facing the future: A guide for parents of young people who have sexually abused*. Russell House Publishing.

Hackett, S., Balfe, M., Masson, H., & Phillips, J. (2014). Family responses to young people who have sexually abused: Anger, ambivalence and acceptance. *Children & Society*, 28(2), 128–139.

Hackett, S., Branigan, P., & Holmes, D. (2019). *Harmful Sexual Behaviour Framework: An evidence-informed operational framework for children and young people displaying harmful sexual behaviours* (2nd edn). NSPCC.

Hackett, S., Phillips, J., Masson, H., & Balfe, M. (2013). Individual, family and abuse characteristics of 700 British child and adolescent sexual abusers. *Child Abuse Review*, 22(4), 232–245.

McCartan, K., Anning, A., & Qureshi, E. (2021). *The impact of sibling sexual abuse on adults who were harmed as children*. UWE, Bristol Research Report.

Sanderson, C. (2006). *Counselling adult survivors of child sexual abuse* (3rd edn). Jessica Kingsley Publishers.

Sanderson, C. (2013). *Counselling skills for working with trauma*. Jessica Kingsley Publishers.

Sanderson, C. (2015). *Counselling skills for working with shame*. Jessica Kingsley Publishers.

Sanderson, C. (2022). *The warrior within: A One in Four handbook to aid recovery for survivors of childhood sexual abuse and violence* (4th edn). One in Four.

Yates, P. (2017). Sibling sexual abuse: Why don't we talk about it? *Journal of Clinical Nursing*, 26(15–16), 2482–2494.

Yates, P., & Allardyce, S. (2021). *Sibling sexual abuse: Knowledge and practice*. Centre of Expertise on Child Sexual Abuse.

Yates, P., & Allardyce, S. (2022). Abuse at the heart of the family: The challenges and complexities of sibling sexual abuse. In K. Uzieblo, W.J. Smid, & K. McCartan (eds), *Challenges in the Management of People Convicted of a Sexual Offence*. Palgrave Macmillan.

CHAPTER 3

Typical Sexual Development and Sexual Behaviour in Children and Young People

Not all sexual interactions between young children are harmful or abusive, and it is essential that parents and professionals know what is considered to be developmentally typical or normative psychosexual development. This chapter will examine developmentally typical sexual behaviour across three major age groups (0–4, 5–12, and 13–18) to increase awareness and understanding of developmentally normative psychosexual development and sexual behaviour in children and young people. Equipped with this, parents and professionals will be able to distinguish between age appropriate consensual sexual activity and harmful sexual behaviour in children and young people.

Children's natural curiosity about their world and people in it, including their own bodies, whether running or jumping or writing, is essential to learning. The development of sexuality in children is one component of their general development, in which they acquire knowledge about their own bodies and those of others through self-exploration, auto-stimulation, comparing themselves to others, and exploring the bodies of others through touch. In this they learn about their bodies, imitate adult behaviours, and experiment with gender roles through sexual play as a way of rehearsing later adult sexuality.

To help professionals and families to understand, identify, and respond to sexual behaviour displayed in children, the UK sexual health charity Brook's provides a traffic light system to distinguish between developmentally safe and healthy sexual behaviours and those that are a cause for concern (see Table 3.1 below). This tool consists of three levels of sexual behaviour in children and young people that professionals can use to identify and respond appropriately when working with children and young people.

The Brook's Sexual Behaviours Traffic Light Tool (licensed and adapted from True Relationships and Reproductive Health, Australia, www.true.org.au/education) identifies three levels of sexual behaviour. 'Green' behaviours are considered to be safe and healthy, and sexually developmentally appropriate in that they represent young children's natural curiosity and experimentation. 'Amber' behaviours are somewhat outside of safe and sexual behaviour in that they are unusual in terms of type of activity, frequency, and duration, and as such may be of potential concern. 'Red' behaviours fall outside of safe and healthy sexual behaviour in that they involve coercion, degrading and threatening behaviour, and significant age and power differences.

In order to identify whether sexual behaviour between children and siblings is aligned with typical sexual development and sexual play, it is essential to distinguish between consensual sexual experimentation and harmful sexual behaviour. This necessitates an understanding of what is generally considered to be age appropriate sexual behaviour and consensual sexual curiosity and experimentation, and what is considered to be non-consensual atypical sexual behaviour.

This is especially the case in SSA to prevent normalising or minimising SSA, and to ensure that sibling sexual experimentation is non-abusive or harmful, rather than assuming such activity is merely sexual experimentation (Yates, 2020). Such knowledge enables parents and professionals to be more aware of a sibling who may be experiencing sexual abuse, or a sibling who may be engaging in harmful sexual behaviour, and who may pose a risk to not just other siblings but also other children. Early detection of HSB towards siblings promotes both protection of the sibling being harmed and support for the harming sibling.

In distinguishing between age appropriate, typical sexual behaviour and atypical sexual behaviour in children, professionals also need to be mindful of differences in sexual behaviour between neurotypical children and those who are neuroatypical, or neurodivergent, and understand their behaviour within the context of neurodiversity rather than shaming the child.

While sexual expression, self-stimulation, and masturbation are typical in the sexual development of children, there are some cultures and religions which do not approve of sexual expression in children.

Socio-cultural factors in terms of values, norms, and expectation are reflected in the family and in interpersonal experiences and act as a powerful force on the child in terms of what is considered to be acceptable or age appropriate behaviour, including sexual prohibitions, sexual shame, and attitudes towards the display of sexuality, and how these can lead to restrictions on sexual behaviour which can shape the sexual development of children as well as their capacity to make meaning of their experiences. While practitioners need to acknowledge cultural differences in the expression of sexuality, they also need to be aware of parental responses in order to respond to children's emerging sexuality and how shame and secrecy can increase the risk and vulnerability to HSB.

Psychosexual Development

Sexual development in children is predicated on the complex interplay between anatomical, biological, physiological, hormonal, cognitive, behavioural, and emotional and socio-cultural factors. These factors are further influenced by family, society, culture, religion, historical time, and exposure to sexual abuse in childhood, all of which shape attitudes towards sexuality, and in turn condition sexual motivation, sexual behaviour, sexual identity, gender, and sense of self. In addition, psychosexual development needs to be understood within the context of physical development as well as sexual knowledge and sexual behaviour, and that children can engage in sexual behaviour without knowledge or understanding of sex or sexuality.

The capacity for sensual arousal and sexual excitation is present in utero and at birth, with male babies capable of reflex erections (Sanderson, 2004). Such reactions are primarily physiological, reflexive responses when feeding, sucking, urinating, and defecating, and from genital stimulation during nappy changes. While initially erotically neutral they become associated with soothing sensual experiences through closeness, satisfaction, and pleasure. These initially indiscriminate sensual reactions become more selectively focused on specific erotic cues or direct stimulation of the breasts or genitals as the child develops and matures. Although some of these early reflexive responses result in orgasm, this is not the primary goal and it is unclear how frequently they occur (Sanderson, 2004). These tend to be involuntary and happen outside conscious awareness or control.

Children are naturally curious about their own and others' bodies. As they explore and touch their own bodies and those of others, they begin to experiment with peers through play. Such sexual play is considered typical sexual development when it is balanced with interest and curiosity about other parts of the child's universe, and is spontaneous and mutual. Healthy sexual exploration is exciting, slightly mischievous and sometimes feels funny and is experienced as fun, full of gaiety, giggles, and laughter, and if discovered and instructed to stop, the children will happily do so and play something else. In addition, typical sexual experimentation occurs between children in mixed gender groups, of similar age and physical size, who are friends rather than siblings.

This is in contrast to being coerced or forced into sexual activity to the exclusion of any other type of play, and where there is an age, size, or power differential, or the relationship between the child and the peer outside of the sexual activity is suffused with hostility or aggression. Such sexual activity, rather than fun, feels confusing and is accompanied by fear, anxiety, guilt, and a deep sense of shame (see Table 3.2).

Sexual Development and Sexual Behaviour in PreSchool Children (0–4)

Babies and young children are able to experience pleasurable sensations when their genitals are stimulated which result in physiological arousal and reflexes such as penile erections in males and reflexive lubrication in females. These are not experienced as 'sexual'; rather they are reflexes which are biologically programmed to elicit pleasure when touching the genital area. It is important to recognise that the child in exploring their body may initially accidentally discover that they can experience pleasure from touching their genitals, which they subsequently want to experience again (Baldwin & Baldwin, 2012) . At this stage the child has little or no sexual knowledge, although they will have limited language for body parts including the genitals, and be inquisitive about their own and other people's bodies such as breasts and genitals, as well as adult sexual behaviour.

The development of sexual behaviour in this stage is mediated through play in which curiosity promotes information gathering about the world, in order to understand and construct meaning. In the first two years of life, play is primarily solitary and focused on self-discovery through autoerotic self-stimulation, to ascertain what is pleasure rather than sexual. Between 6 and 12 months babies discover that when certain parts of the body are touched, exposed to the air, or stimulated, pleasant sensations occur. Initially this is discovered by accident, such as during nappy changing, and because pleasurable sensations are elicited, it is more likely to be repeated (Sanderson, 2004). While such sensual pleasure is experienced as soothing and comforting, the extent to which it is repeated will depend on whether parents or primary caregivers negatively or positively reinforce accidental touching or self-exploration.

Between two and five years children become increasingly more social, and their peer interactions increase; they move from being autoerotic to becoming socio-sexual (Sanderson, 2004). There is an increased interest in bathroom activities and the use of language to describe body parts, including the genitals and lavatorial functions. Children at this age often poke or squeeze the breasts of adult females, accompanied by laughter or running away in delight. They may also take pleasure in taking off all their clothes or display their genitals to others, especially in boys who take delight in displaying their erections. Once children gain increased muscle and motor control, and gain more dexterity, around the age of two and a half, they may simulate masturbation either by using their own hands, or by rubbing their genitals with stuffed toys, blankets, dolls, or arms of chairs, or by rhythmically thrusting the genitals against objects.

Sexual activities increasingly involve interactions with others which include kissing, hugging, touching, using rude words, and telling rude jokes, although these are often sporadic, and fairly cursory and superficial. The most common sexual play at this stage consists of imitating the behaviour of adults and traditionally consisted of playing 'mummies and daddies' and lying on top of each other while fully clothed. If unclothed, the sexual activity tends to be confined to showing each other their genitals rather than fondling each other's genitals or sticking fingers or objects into the vagina, or anal cavity. As well as being less usual to insert fingers or objects, if this hurts they quickly desist.

Table 3.2 Summary of sexual development and typical sexual behaviour in preschool children (0–4)

Sexual development	Typical sexual behaviour
Limited peer contact	Autoerotic
Solitary play	Self-exploration
Curiosity about their body	Self-stimulation

Touching of genitals – increases when tired, distressed, or going to sleep	Touches or rubs own genitals
	Watches others' bodies
	Squeezes females' breasts
Genital pleasure and comfort	Looks at genitals
Increasing awareness of gender	Shows off genitals, especially erections
Interest in anatomical differences	Interested in bathroom functions
Interest in differences between child, teen, and adult bodies	Uses childish dirty language to talk about body parts
Curiosity how babies are made and where they come from	Lavatorial language
Associate genitals with urination and bowel movement	Imitative pretend play of observed adult behaviour: 'mummies and daddies', or 'doctors and nurses'
Increased social-sexual play	Inserts objects into orifices but stops if painful
	Squeezes females' breasts and bottoms or genitals of adults
	Enjoys being naked

Sexual Development and Sexual Behaviour in School Age Children (5–12)

During this stage there are significant physical changes as children grow and mature. Some children also experience hormonal changes, with some eight- and nine-year-old children entering puberty and developing secondary sex characteristics. Some girls will start menstruating and develop breasts, whereas some boys will experience changes in their genitalia and the tonal quality of their voice. This is accompanied with an increased sexual awakening and more conscious awareness of sexual feelings, and gender and sexual identity. Towards the end of this stage there is an increase in sexual fantasies which tend to be accompanied by nocturnal emissions ('wet dreams') and masturbation.

Throughout this stage there is an increase in knowledge about sex, sexual behaviour, and sexual acts, largely acquired from peers, social media, and TV and films. Older children become more adept at simulating intercourse, kissing, petting with peers, with some engaging in full intercourse without awareness of the consequences of this, or being able to give informed consent. There is also an increase in the use of sexual language and the use of slang words for genitals. As most of this information is derived from peers there is often considerable confusion and misinformation which can be anxiety provoking. As children become more self-conscious and self-aware they crave more privacy around their bodies and feel less comfortable with displays of public nudity, and tend to masturbate in private rather than in public.

During this stage most children will have had their first socio-sexual experience through games such as spin the bottle or strip poker (Sanderson, 2004). Although the erotic and sexual intent increases as the child gets older, sexual play nevertheless remains a sporadic activity and does not necessarily increase with the approach of puberty. As masturbation becomes less random and more sexually specific, children discover increasingly creative ways of masturbating. Girls discover that water stimulation through directing a waterspout or showerhead at their vagina in the bath feels good, while boys find that climbing and shimmying down poles feels good on their penis. This information is usually shared with peers and friends, which gives rise to further experimentation. Nevertheless, there are still periods of inhibition and dis-inhibition (see Table 3.3).

Towards the end of this stage a significant number of children will have been exposed to pornography, with some watching it regularly. This is often driven by peers who often encourage others to watch pornography within group settings, or post and share sexual images with each other. Despite the increased exposure to sexual behaviour there is a lack of knowledge of the role of intimacy in relationships. This lack of knowledge and reduced capacity to process the full meaning of sexual behaviour leaves some children vulnerable to either being sexually abused or to sexually harming other children.

In some cases, peers may coerce others to take sexualised images of their siblings to share on social media, while others may attempt to re-enact what they have seen online with younger children or siblings.

Table 3.3 Summary of sexual development and typical sexual behaviour in school age children (5–12)

Sexual development	Typical sexual behaviour
Physical growth and bodily changes	Increase in consensual experimental interaction
Increased peer contact	Touches self – more specific focus on genitals
Other children may bring up new ideas about sex	Increase in kissing, touching, showing holding hands

Increased need for privacy while bathing and undressing	Repulsed by or drawn to opposite gender or same gender
Towards end of this stage sense of modesty develops	Asks more questions about masturbation, pregnancy, sexual behaviour
Increased awareness of private and public behaviour	Talks about sex more
	Increased use of sexual language
More self-conscious, inhibited about body	Tells dirty jokes
	Exhibitionistic behaviour such as mooning
Towards end of stage, pubertal hormonal changes	Watches pornography
	Posts and shares sexual images
Menstruation in girls	Sexting
Genital and voice changes in boys	Dating
	Petting
Secondary sex characteristics	Simulates sexual intercourse
Nocturnal emissions	Vaginal or anal intercourse in pre-adolescents
Sexual fantasies	
Intentional, focused masturbation	Solitary masturbation
	Increased need for privacy around own body
	Consensual kissing, hugging, holding hands with peers

Sexual Development and Behaviour in Adolescents (13–18)

Most children and young people will enter puberty in this stage and will have experienced hormonal changes and the development of secondary sex characteristics, as well as fluctuations in emotional reactions. As the sex organs mature there is an increase in sexual feelings and heightened sexual arousal, which is often accompanied by exploration around gender and sexual identity and sexual orientation (see Table 3.4). There is an increase in 'locker room' behaviour in which young males share sexual fantasies and sexual prowess, or engage in masturbation competitions to see who can ejaculate first, or the furthest, or the most. In contrast, females compare breast size and their figures with others, especially through social media. This can have detrimental effects if they feel they do not fit into a socially accepted ideal which can give rise to a range of mental health difficulties, or body modification through cosmetic surgery.

Intense sexual feelings often result in crushes on same sex or opposite sex peers or adult role models such as teachers, sporting heroes, or celebrity figures as a way to channel the heightened sexual arousal. To manage sexual arousal many adolescents turn to watching pornography, and while this can lead to an increase in sexual knowledge of sexual practices, it does not enhance knowledge with regard to intimacy and relationships. This can lead to romantic relationship difficulties which become predicated on sexual behaviour rather than relationship skills. Increasingly young people also access online sexual contact which can render them vulnerable to sextortion.

Some adolescents begin dating, which involves open mouth kissing, petting (under and over clothes), touching each other's genitals, simulating intercourse, vaginal or anal stimulation, oral sex, or mutual masturbation. Much of this is conducted privately, although kissing and petting competitions in groups can and do take place. These experiences may subsequently be recounted to other peers to impress, or involve sharing intimate photos. Self-discovery and observation still primarily determines many of these activities, although young people towards the end of this stage do take this sexual activity further. Depending on cultural, moral, religious, or health restrictions, penile genital contact may be avoided although oral sex or anal sex may be indulged in. Increases in such activity, including full sexual intercourse, will become more predominant as the young person matures.

Table 3.4 Summary of sexual development and typical sexual behaviour in adolescents (13–18)

Characteristics	Typical sexual behaviour
Hormonal changes	Asks questions about relationships and sexual behaviour
Menstruation in females	
Development of secondary sex characteristics	Uses sexual language
	Talks about sexual acts with peers
More self-conscious about body and body changes	Watches pornography
	Uses online sexual services
Increased need for privacy around the body	Masturbates in private
	Experiments sexually with same age peers
Mood swings	
Confusion about body changes	Consensual sexual exploration and petting
Doubts around sexuality	

Exploration of gender and sexual identity	Consensual vaginal and anal exploration
	Mutual masturbation
Exploration of sexual orientation	Consensual oral sex
Fears about relationships	Consensual full sexual intercourse
Fears of getting pregnant	Consensual and private sexting and sharing of intimate images
Fears around contracting STIs	
Anxieties about being attractive and finding partners	Sexual jokes
	Having sexual and non-sexual relationships

In knowing what is considered to be developmentally typical sexual behaviour in children and young people, it is necessary to be apprised of what is deemed to be developmentally atypical sexual behaviour and what can lead to HSB and SSA. The next chapter will examine the range of HSB and developmentally atypical sexual behaviour, and how this manifests across the three age groups. It will also highlight the range of sexual behaviours in children and young people with learning difficulties, and those who are neurodivergent, and examine to what extent these children are at risk of being sexually abused or displaying problematic or harmful behaviours.

Further Reading

Caffaro, J. (2020). Sibling abuse of other children. In R. Geffner, V. Vieth, V. Vaughan-Eden, A. Rosenbaum, L. Hamberger, & J. White (eds), *Handbook of Interpersonal Violence across the Lifespan*. Springer.

Caffaro, J.V., & Conn-Caffaro, A. (1998). *Sibling abuse trauma: Assessment and intervention strategies for children, families and adults*. Routledge.

Hackett, S. (2001). *Facing the future: A guide for parents of young people who have sexually abused*. Russell House Publishing.

Hackett, S. (2004). *What works for children and young people with harmful sexual behaviours?* Barnardo's.

Hackett, S. (2010). Children and young people with harmful sexual behaviours. In C. Barter, & D. Berridge (eds), *Children behaving badly? Peer violence between children and young people*. Wiley-Blackwell.

Hackett, S., Balfe, M., Masson, H., & Phillips, J. (2014). Family responses to young people who have sexually abused: Anger, ambivalence and acceptance. *Children & Society*, 28(2), 128–139.

Hackett, S., Branigan, P., & Holmes, D. (2019). *Harmful Sexual Behaviour Framework: An evidence-informed operational framework for children and young people displaying harmful sexual behaviours* (2nd edn). NSPCC.

Hackett, S., Phillips, J., Masson, H., & Balfe, M. (2013). Individual, family and abuse characteristics of 700 British child and adolescent sexual abusers. *Child Abuse Review*, 22(4), 232–245.

McCartan, K., Anning, A., & Qureshi, E. (2021). *The impact of sibling sexual abuse on adults who were harmed as children*. UWE, Bristol Research Report.

Punch, S. (2008). 'You can do nasty things to your brothers and sisters without a reason': Siblings' backstage behaviour. *Children & Society*, 22(5), 333–344.

Sanderson, C. (2004). *The seduction of children: Empowering parents and teachers to protect children from sexual abuse*. Jessica Kingsley Publishers.

Sanderson, C. (2022). *The warrior within: A One in Four handbook to aid recovery for survivors of childhood sexual abuse and violence* (4th edn). One in Four.

White, N., & Hughes, C. (2018). *Why siblings matter: The role of brother and sister relationships in development and well-being*. Routledge.

Yates, P., & Allardyce, S. (2021). *Sibling sexual abuse: Knowledge and practice*. Centre of Expertise on Child Sexual Abuse.

Yates, P., & Allardyce, S. (2022). Abuse at the heart of the family: The challenges and complexities of sibling sexual abuse. In K. Uzieblo, W.J. Smid, & K. McCartan (eds), *Challenges in the Management of People Convicted of a Sexual Offence*. Palgrave Macmillan.

CHAPTER 4

Atypical Sexual Behaviour in Children and Young People

This chapter will examine what is considered to be developmentally atypical sexual behaviour and how this manifests across the three age groups and manifests in HSB and SSA. It will also explore the range of sexual behaviours in children and young people with learning difficulties, and those who are neurodivergent, and examine to what extent these children are at risk of being sexually abused or displaying problematic or harmful behaviours.

Atypical Sexual Behaviour
In understanding what is considered to be developmentally typical sexual behaviour in children, professionals are more able to distinguish this from atypical sexual behaviour and what is considered cause for concern. The risk of developmentally inappropriate sexual behaviour is elevated when there is unequal power due to age, size, cognitive knowledge, status, authority, or privilege. Commonly the relationship between siblings lacks mutuality with very few interactions or play, other than sexualised games.

Children and young people who display atypical sexual behaviour have a heightened preoccupation with sex, and as a result feel compelled to engage in repetitive sexualised behaviour to the exclusion of other forms of play, and find it hard to desist when instructed to. The qualitative nature of the sexual behaviour is also significantly different to typical sexual behaviour as it is often pre-planned, ritualistic and involves actual penetration of the vagina and anus with objects, toys, fingers, or penis, even when it hurts. Often this sort of sexual exploration is accompanied by coercion, threats, force or violence, or deception, manipulation, bribery or gifts, or special attention to ensure secrecy and silence.

The obsessive nature inherent in developmentally atypical sexual behaviour is also demonstrated in compulsive masturbation, often performed in public, as well as heightened levels of sexual exhibitionism and voyeurism.

In order to set up opportunities to engage in sexual behaviour the child tends to seek out the company of young children or younger siblings and spend unusual amounts of time with them. They may insist on hugging or kissing them even when the child doesn't want to, or expose their genitals to them. Some may take younger children or siblings to 'secret' places or hideaways to play 'special' age inappropriate games with them, or force sex on them. Alternatively, they may show the younger child sexual abuse images and pornography or ply them with alcohol or drugs.

Atypical Sexual Behaviour in Children Aged 0–4

Children are curious about their bodies from birth and instinctively want to explore their bodies and the bodies of others. This developmentally appropriate behaviour can be hijacked if the child has experienced CSA, trauma, or ACEs, or lives in chaotic and unstable family environments. Common signs of developmentally atypical sexual behaviour include obsessive preoccupation with sexual play to the exclusion of all other types of play and which lacks spontaneity as it is often pre-planned and ritualised (see Box 4.1). In addition the child is not easily distracted away from sexual play and does not stop sexual interactions when requested to. While masturbation is normal in this age group, excessive public masturbation, exhibitionism, or voyeurism can indicate atypical sexual expression. If the sexual interactions and behaviour involves coercion, threats, secrecy, or use of force and control, or involves injury to self or others, this would indicate cause for concern.

> Box 4.1 Atypical sexual behaviour in children aged 0–4
>
> - Engages in adult-like sexual contact with other children
> - Displays adult-like sexual knowledge

- Relates to adults and children in a sexual manner
- Frequently rubs themselves sexually against others despite being asked not to
- Compulsive genital touching or masturbation
- Forces sexual contact on other children
- Does not stop masturbation or sexual play when asked to
- Inserts objects into orifices even if painful
- Preoccupied with sexual behaviour and activities
- Only wants to engage in sexual play to the exclusion of any other play activity
- Acts out adult-type sexual behaviour with toys or objects
- Open mouthed kissing
- Knowledge of taste, texture, and smell of semen
- Uses sexually explicit language
- Discusses sexual acts
- Pulling other children's skirts up/pants or trousers down
- Following others into the lavatory or changing room to look at them, or touch them
- Persistent touching of genitals of other children and adults
- Talking about sexual activities seen online or on TV
- Preoccupied with adult sexual behaviour

Atypical Sexual Behaviour in Children Aged 5–12

As children become more self-conscious about their bodies, especially as they come into puberty, they tend to be more private and less preoccupied with exploratory sexual play. Children who continue to be preoccupied with sexual experimentation or sexually interact with much younger children involving oral, vaginal, or anal penetration using fingers, penis, or objects, or enforce genital kissing, would be considered to be engaging in atypical sexual behaviour (see Box 4.2). The excessive use of pornography, including illegal pornography or viewing child abuse images or websites, would also be a cause for concern especially if they then attempted to re-enact these with younger siblings, or other children.

Box 4.2 Atypical sexual behaviour in children aged 5–12

- Masturbates in public
- Compulsive masturbation
- Forces sexual activity on other children, especially younger children
- Non-consensual sexual experimentation
- Displays adult sexual behaviour
- Shows adult sexual knowledge
- Knows smell, texture, and taste of semen
- Preoccupation with sexual behaviour and activity
- Relates to adults and children in sexual manner
- Does not stop sexual behaviour when asked to
- Sources and views online pornography
- Posts sexual images as a way of humiliating and shaming others
- Engages in TA-HSB
- Displays problematic and harmful sexual behaviour
- Sexual violence and rape
- Sadistic sexual behaviour
- Preoccupation with sex such as sex talk, images, play, or artwork
- Repeatedly asks questions about sex, even after answers have been supplied
- Verbal, physical, or cyber-sexual bullying, face to face or online
- Mutual masturbation
- LGBT targeted bullying
- Exhibitionism (flashing, mooning)
- Attempts oral or penetrative sex
- Risky sexual behaviour or sharing contact details online
- Worrying about being pregnant or STIs

Atypical Sexual Behaviour in Teenagers aged 13–18

While there is a normative surge of sexual interest in this age group partly due to puberty, hormonal changes, and the development of secondary sex characteristics, there are certain atypical sexual behaviours that can be deemed problematic or sexually harmful. These include any sexual interactions involving children younger than themselves, or the use of coercion, force, control, domination, or humiliation. Any non-consensual sexual activity such as attempts to touch or expose others' genitals without permission, exhibiting genitals to others, exerting sexual pressure on others, sexual harassment, and stalking is indicative of problematic sexual behaviour (see Box 4.3).

TA-HSB involving sexual themes of degrading others, or sharing unsolicited sexual images of themselves or others, are forms of HSB, as is any non-consensual forced sexual contact, rape, or sexual assault.

Paul

Twelve-year-old Paul, a later developer, was desperate to fit in with his peers and would often go along with whatever they wanted him to do. He felt they were beginning to accept him as they allowed him to watch pornography on their phones which he found arousing. After a few months his peers suggested that as he had a younger sister he should get her to pose naked for him and take photos to send to the peer group. Paul felt uncomfortable about this but complied as he feared he would be excluded from the peer group. He suggested to his sister that they play a game with forfeits which meant she had to take off items of clothing. His sister thought this was great fun, until Paul started to film this and send the images to his friends.

Box 4.3 Atypical sexual behaviour in teenagers aged 13–18

- Masturbates in public
- Uses aggressive sexual language
- Sexual harassment
- Sends sexually abusive texts
- Revenge porn
- Sextortion
- Engages in TA-HSB
- Engages in HSB and sexual violence
- Non-consensual sex and rape
- Drug-induced rape
- Excessive use of exploitative or violent pornography

- Looks at child abuse images
- Sexual contact with much younger children or siblings
- Concern about body image
- Risky behaviour such as giving out contact details online, meeting up through online contact alone
- Exposing self to others, voyeurism, mooning, obscene behaviour and gestures
- Taking and sending naked or sexually provocative images of self or others
- Compulsive preoccupation with sex, to the exclusion of other daily activities
- Compulsive masturbation or compulsive sexual behaviour
- Engaging in ChemSex (sexual activity while under the influence of drugs such as methamphetamine or mephedrone, typically involving multiple participants)
- Joining adult-only sexual networking sites and falsifying personal information
- Sexual degradation and humiliation of self and others
- Sexually aggressive/exploitative behaviour
- Use of power and control in sexual relationships
- Genital injury to self and others
- Sexual activity with family members
- Sexually explicit talk with younger children
- Sexual contact with others where there is a significant age difference, younger or older, or those in authority
- Involvement in sexual exploitation, sexual trafficking, or gang sexual violence
- Sexual activity with animals
- Transactional sex, trading money or gifts for sex, face to face or on 'OnlyFans' sites

Compulsive masturbation and excessive preoccupation with pornography or use of online sex websites may also be a cause for concern and needs to be monitored.

Wanda

Wanda came from a family where anything to do with sex or nudity was taboo and could never be talked about. Unbeknownst to the family, Wanda's older brother Samuel had been fascinated by online sexual images and began watching pornography from a young age. As he entered puberty his use of pornography became more and more excessive and he would spend a considerable part of the evening online. As masturbating to these images became less and less satisfying, he began to coerce Wanda to copy some of the sexual acts he had seen, which over time culminated in full penetrative sex. As Samuel found this considerably more satisfying than masturbating he continued to regularly sexually abuse Wanda until he left home.

Sexual Development and Sexual Behaviour in Neurodivergent Children

Typical sexual development and sexual behaviour is seen in all children especially with regard to exploring their bodies and other bodies, looking and touching, sexual excitation, masturbation, and consensual sexual activity. Professionals and parents need to be aware, however, that the sexual development and sexual behaviour in some neurodivergent children with autism spectrum disorder (ASD) or severe learning disabilities can differ from neurotypical children. This is primarily due to sensory hyper- or hypo-sensitivities, repetitive behaviours, narrow range of interests, as well as communication and social skills difficulties in understanding how other people think and feel, or how their behaviour impacts other people.

Professionals also need to be aware that neurodivergent children are more at risk of being sexually abused and that some of the non-normative sexual behaviour may be re-enactments of the abuse experience which needs to be assessed and processed through specialist therapeutic support. While neurodivergent children are more at risk of CSA, practitioners need to be mindful and not assume that any problematic or HSB is a direct result of a history of sexual abuse.

While most neurodivergent children are not a cause for concern, some may unwittingly display problematic or HSB. Such children require clear guidance with regard to appropriate and not appropriate physical and sexual boundaries. Denoting inappropriate sexual behaviour as 'amusing' or 'cute' can have a significant effect on the child's developing sexual identity as they grow, and create anxiety in the future.

Problematic sexual behaviour in neurodivergent children and young people is often characterised by persistently showing their genitals or bottom or touching their own genitals in public, or following or frequently contacting someone they like. In some cases this can result in HSB wherein they might force, coerce, or threaten a younger child or sibling to take part in sexual touching.

Sensory hyper- or hypo-sensitivities in neurodivergent children often cluster around seeking out or avoiding certain sensory experiences, especially involving touch and taste, as well as things to see, or hear. Many children and young people with ASD touch other people's clothing or hair, or rub their arms, legs, or genitals against objects or people, or engage in cuddling, mouth to mouth kissing, or sitting on people's lap that they don't really know.

The narrowing of interest and repetitive behaviours associated with ASD can result in focusing on specific sexual behaviour or fetishising sexual parts by stroking or staring for prolonged periods of time at people's breasts or buttocks without understanding how that might be seen as sexual or distressing to the other person. This can render some ASD children more vulnerable to repetitive and ritualistic sexual behaviour including compulsive masturbation.

Social skills difficulties include communication deficits and not being able to read other people's thoughts, feelings, body language, facial expressions, tone of voice, or behavioural cues. This can result in misinterpreting friendliness as flirtation or sexual interest, and expressing sexual thoughts aloud. Some may have unrealistic sexual expectations from watching sexual content in films or pornography, or misperceive that if they want to have sex the other person will also want to, which can lead to unwanted sexual advances. In addition, they may not understand what is considered appropriate behaviour in private and public places and thus touch or expose their genitals, or masturbate in public.

Children and Young People with Learning Difficulties

Some children and young people with learning difficulties, or who face mental and physical challenges such as Down syndrome, can display problematic or harmful sexual behaviour. This can range from inappropriate or compulsive masturbation, touching, and sexualised language, to stalking, rape, and risky online behaviours such as accessing illegal forms of pornography or viewing child sexual abuse images. As children with learning difficulties are more susceptible to CSA, it is essential to assess whether they have been sexually abused or have additional mental health needs. Research has shown that children with disabilities are less likely to be put on the child protection register and less likely to receive therapeutic interventions, rendering them more at risk of going on to sexually abuse other children, including siblings.

> ### Hailey
> Hailey and her brother John both had learning difficulties. When Hailey disclosed that John was trying to insert his penis into her and make her do things she didn't like, the initial professional response was that Hailey must have got it wrong, allowing John to continue to sexually abuse her for several more months. When it was finally discovered that John was sexually harming Hailey, it was minimised in terms of intent given their learning difficulties, with neither child receiving appropriate therapeutic support.

While children and young people with learning difficulties often have a healthy interest in sexuality they often lack knowledge of what is considered appropriate sexual behaviour. This can be due to lack of sexual knowledge, cognitive capacity which limits understanding of the expression of sexual needs, the role of consent, lack of sexual experience, and lack of social and communication skills with regard to physical and sexual boundaries, difficulties in separating private from public, safe from risky behaviours, and appropriate from inappropriate sexual encounters (Frawley & Wilson, 2016), as well as difficulties in asserting themselves when exposed to HSB due to physical or motor limitations.

Some children with severe learning difficulties or who face mental or physical challenges find specific objects or textures sexually arousing and seek them out for stimulation. Self-stimulation such as touching or rubbing genitals against objects or people is part of typical sexual development in young children which can become problematic in children with learning disabilities. They may compensate for lack of non-sexual stimulation, or boredom, with masturbation becoming a substitute, or touching or engaging inappropriate physical and sexual play with younger siblings. Alternatively, they may engage younger siblings in watching pornography and ask them to act out what they have seen online. If there is reduced cognitive or intellectual capacity they may not realise that SSA or HSB is both harmful to them and others.

Further frustration can occur due to physical difficulties in getting erections, being able to masturbate or ejaculate, or due to psychotropic medication. Such difficulties can create shame and anxieties around sex, leading to secretive and furtive sexual behaviour and an increased vulnerability to sexual abuse. Professionals and parents need to be aware of these factors alongside psychosocial factors such as gender, race, and culture and how these intersect with regard to problematic sexual behaviour or HSB, and respond appropriately in supporting parents and neurodivergent children.

Sexual Behaviour in Children Who Have Been Sexually Abused

Children who have experienced premature sexualisation through sexual abuse often become sexually preoccupied due to sexual over-stimulation which they are unable to integrate or make sense of. This can result in acting out developmentally advanced sexual behaviour, and a preoccupation with sexual themes in their play activities. While this may represent unconscious attempts to alert others to the sexual abuse, it also reflects confusion, shame, and anxiety about sex. Some children may use sexual behaviour as a way to relate to others and will engage in sexual activity as a way of connecting. While sexual stimulation can be a form of self-soothing behaviour, sexually abused children feel no delight in their bodies and do not see sexual activity as fun or lighthearted. Instead they experience sex as arousing yet confusing, fearful and something they feel compelled to do. Many sexually abused children dissociate during the sexual activity and show little or no emotion either during or after the sexual activity.

As a consequence of the sexual abuse, their sexual behaviour is significantly different to what is seen in typical sexual development and can range from hyper-sexual excitation to avoidance of anything associated with the body or nudity. Children with hyper-sexual excitation are more sexually sensitised and often feel compelled to seek out sexual stimulation, either autoerotically, or with others. This can lead to compulsive masturbation in which the child seeks comfort, but it may be so intense and persistent as to cause abrasions and lesions to the genitals. They may also engage in more sophisticated and adult-like sexual behaviours, including oral sex, forcible penetration of objects into the vagina and anus, and vaginal and anal sexual intercourse. This hyper-sexualised behaviour differs significantly from typical sexual behaviour which is more sporadic, spontaneous, and less obsessive.

In contrast, sexually abused children who become hypo-sexual will tend to withdraw and avoid all physical contact and become fearful or distressed when hugged or touched, or when having to remove their clothes, bathing, or have their nappy changed. They may neglect personal hygiene, or refuse to change their underwear as a way to ward off potential sexual attention.

Atypical Sexual Behaviour Associated with SSA

Not all sibling sexual behaviour is harmful and it is not uncommon for younger siblings to engage in sexual exploration and experimentation which are age appropriate (Johnson, 2015). These are often mutually initiated and can emerge from sexual games which can in some cases become coercive (Tener, 2019). In addition, the extent to which both siblings consent to the sexual activity can vary on different occasions and change over time (Tener et al., 2017) and is dependent on the nature of their relationship outside the sexual activity. This is particularly the case where siblings may be drawn together for comfort and support due to other abuse or stress in the family, and which then becomes sexualised.

The sexualised behaviour in SSA is much more frequent and ritualised than in age appropriate sexual behaviour and can develop into a pattern of sexual activity which can persist over many years. Atypical sexual behaviour associated with SSA is when an older sibling prefers spending unusual amounts of time with a younger sibling, or one that they have power or control over, which is generally misconstrued as loving and caring behaviour. They will often engage in 'special' games, often in 'secret' places, that are not appropriate for either sibling. There may be an insistence on hugging and kissing even if the sibling doesn't want to. The nature of the sexual activity escalates over time, starting with playing games which are fun and consensual, which then become progressively more sexualised. This is confusing as, although the younger sibling has agreed to play the non-sexualised game, they are drawn into sexualised activity which they are not able to consent to and yet feel complicit in.

In some cases of SSA, the older sibling ignores the young sibling and spends little time playing with them other than as a prelude to HSB. The younger sibling is so delighted when the harming sibling shows any interest in them or wishes to 'play a game' with them that they are happy to go along with whatever they are instructed to do, as they fear the consequences of not complying. This is the antithesis of mutual sexual experimentation as it is suffused with fear, anxiety, secrecy, and shame. In addition, some siblings may show sexual content to a younger sibling such as pornography and suggest they imitate and act out what they have seen. In some cases, especially with older siblings, this might be accompanied with sharing alcohol or drugs as this has a dis-inhibiting effect and may make it harder to remember precisely what happened. For more on harmful sexual behaviour please see Chapter 2.

The impact of SSA and HSB will be examined in the next two chapters, with the next chapter highlighting the impact of SSA. Although much of SSA is normalised, and many siblings report little or no harm at the time of the abuse, it will nevertheless have considerable impact. The next chapter will explore how repeated SSA over a prolonged period of time can lead to complex trauma (C-PTSD) and DTD which can result in a range of trauma reactions, not least emotional dysregulation, prolonged fear states, dissociation, flashbacks, and sleep disturbances, as well as shame, self-blame, and self-harming behaviours. These will be identified and linked to the risk of delayed trauma which can surface later in life.

Further Reading

Caffaro, J. (2020). Sibling abuse of other children. In R. Geffner, V. Vieth, V. Vaughan-Eden, A. Rosenbaum, L. Hamberger, & J. White (eds), *Handbook of Interpersonal Violence across the Lifespan*. Springer.

Caffaro, J.V., & Conn-Caffaro, A. (1998). *Sibling abuse trauma: Assessment and intervention strategies for children, families and adults*. Routledge.

Hackett, S. (2001). *Facing the future: A guide for parents of young people who have sexually abused*. Russell House Publishing.

Hackett, S. (2004). *What works for children and young people with harmful sexual behaviours?* Barnardo's.

Hackett, S. (2010). Children and young people with harmful sexual behaviours. In C. Barter, & D. Berridge (eds), *Children behaving badly? Peer violence between children and young people*. Wiley-Blackwell.

Hackett, S., Balfe, M., Masson, H., & Phillips, J. (2014). Family responses to young people who have sexually abused: Anger, ambivalence and acceptance. *Children & Society, 28*(2), 128–139.

Hackett, S., Branigan, P., & Holmes, D. (2019). *Harmful Sexual Behaviour Framework: An evidence-informed operational framework for children and young people displaying harmful sexual behaviours* (2nd edn). NSPCC.

Hackett, S., Phillips, J., Masson, H., & Balfe, M. (2013). Individual, family and abuse characteristics of 700 British child and adolescent sexual abusers. *Child Abuse Review*, *22*(4), 232–245.

McCartan, K., Anning, A., & Qureshi, E. (2021). *The impact of sibling sexual abuse on adults who were harmed as children*. UWE, Bristol Research Report.

Punch, S. (2008). 'You can do nasty things to your brothers and sisters without a reason': Siblings' backstage behaviour. *Children & Society*, *22*(5), 333–344.

Sanderson, C. (2004). *The seduction of children: Empowering parents and teachers to protect children from sexual abuse*. Jessica Kingsley Publishers.

Sanderson, C. (2022). *The warrior within: A One in Four handbook to aid recovery for survivors of childhood sexual abuse and violence* (4th edn). One in Four.

White, N., & Hughes, C. (2018). *Why siblings matter: The role of brother and sister relationships in development and well-being*. Routledge.

Yates, P., & Allardyce, S. (2021). *Sibling sexual abuse: Knowledge and practice*. Centre of Expertise on Child Sexual Abuse.

Yates, P., & Allardyce, S. (2022). Abuse at the heart of the family: The challenges and complexities of sibling sexual abuse. In K. Uzieblo, W.J. Smid, & K. McCartan (eds), *Challenges in the Management of People Convicted of a Sexual Offence*. Palgrave Macmillan.

CHAPTER 5

The Impact of Sibling Sexual Abuse

This chapter will highlight the impact of SSA and although many siblings report little or no harm at the time of the abuse, it can have considerable impact. Given the proximity of the siblings living under the same roof, and if the SSA is repeated over a prolonged period of time, it can lead to complex trauma (C-PTSD) and DTD which can result in a range of trauma reactions, including toxic stress, emotional dysregulation, prolonged fear states, dissociation, flashbacks, sleep disturbances, as well as shame, self-blame, and self-harming behaviours. These will be identified and linked to the risk of delayed trauma which can surface later in life.

The impact of SSA can vary enormously from child to child, even if the child is not aware of any harm at the time of the sexual contact. Young children are not able fully to understand the effects of sexual interactions between siblings and may believe that sexual touching, stroking, and kissing is normal, fun, exciting, and pleasurable. Even if they do not experience it as abuse or trauma at the time, it nevertheless has the potential to impact on a number of areas of their lives: emotional, cognitive, physical, behavioural, interpersonal, and sexual (see Table 5.1).

Children who have experienced SSA are not able to trust their own perceptions and can no longer trust themselves, or others. This confusion can have damaging effects on the child both short and long term. Doubt and uncertainty, fear and embarrassment, guilt and shame all prevent the child from seeking help from those who could protect them. To cover up their shame and guilt they hide away, shunning peers and closeness with others, including their primary caregiver(s), for fear that the 'secret' will slip out. Their loneliness and isolation reinforces their fear, making them more dependent on the abuser. The child feels trapped with no escape, sentenced to endure the SSA until they are old enough to escape. As the impact of SSA varies from child to child, this chapter will explore how the impact of SSA on the neurobiological development of young children can lead to trauma reactions, as well as PTSD, C-PTSD, DTD, dissociation, and memory deficits.

Most studies indicate that SSA impacts on the child in numerous ways, many of which are harmful (Sanderson, 2004; Caffaro & Conn-Caffaro, 2014; Caffaro, 2020; McCartan et al., 2021). Research has shown that SSA can have significant ongoing lifelong effects (Caffaro & Conn-Caffaro, 2014; Caffaro, 2020; McCartan et al., 2021) although it varies from individual to individual. The impact tends to cluster around emotional dysregulation, PTSD trauma symptoms, attachment and relationship difficulties, changes in sense of self, shame, and self-blame, as well as physical health.

While not all children who have experienced either CSA or SSA will develop trauma reactions, research has shown that 30–40% of children who experience physical or sexual abuse will end up developing PTSD in childhood (Scheeringa, 2011; American Psychiatric Association, 2013). These harmful effects are often underestimated by family and professionals as SSA is often minimised.

The impact of SSA can also result in a range of trauma symptoms such as emotional dysregulation, dissociation, attachment difficulties, changes in sense of self, shame, and self-blame, as well as compromised physical health. Even if the sexual activity is not experienced as abusive it doesn't mean it does not have an impact in the longer term, with children going on to develop delayed trauma reactions when they start dating or entering sexual relationships.

Amelia

Amelia was sexually abused by her older brother for a number of years. Although she had largely forgotten about the sexual abuse, she became plagued by confusing bodily responses when she entered her first sexual relationship. Whenever she became intimate with her partner she found herself freezing, becoming rigid, zoning out, or crying uncontrollably. While initially Amelia was unable to link these responses to what happened with her brother, she started to make a link when she started to have physical and visual memories of the abuse and entered therapy.

Table 5.1 Summary of impact of sibling sexual abuse

Emotional	Cognitive	Behavioural	Physical	Sexual	Interpersonal
Shame and guilt	Poor concentration, attention – focus	Avoidant	Sleep disturbances – nightmares, night terrors	Persistent inappropriate sexual behaviour – children, siblings, adults, toys	Fear of closeness – hugging, cuddling
Self-loathing	Impaired executive functioning – thinking, decision making, impaired learning	Compliant – submissive	Discomfort around body	Sexual themes in art stories, or play	Eroticisation of closeness or anger
Self-conscious		Hostile – aggressive	Somatisation – recurring illness, no medical origin	Adult understanding of sex	Lack of trust in self and others
Self-doubt		Sexualised play			Need to hide – make small, invisible, conceal self
Feel a failure	Dissociation	Regressive behaviour – bedwetting, thumbsucking, clinginess	Itching, inflammation – oral, genital, urethral, anal	Compulsive masturbation	Shyness
Lack of confidence	Disruptions in memory			Compulsive sexual behaviour	
Lack of initiative – self-agency	Denial		Bruises on body, especially genital or buttock areas		Lonely – isolated, alienated, lack of belongingness
Fear		Changes in eating and sleeping patterns		Exhibitionism	Reduced communication skills
Anxiety	Withdrawal into fantasy	Risky behaviours		Voyeurism	
Confusion	Under-/over-achievement in school	Running away		Fear of sex	Inhibited – lack of spontaneity
Powerlessness		Accident prone		Adolescent pregnancy	Role confusion
Helplessness	Cognitive distortions	Self-destructive behaviours			Mind reading
Unlovable		Self-harm		Problematic and harmful sexual behaviour	Over-sensitive to others' needs or moods
Inferiority, worthlessness, inadequacy		Suicide attempts			
Frozenness					Self-sufficient
Anger					

The differential effects of the impact of child SSA can be further compounded if the child experiences sexual arousal such as having an erection, becoming lubricated, or having an orgasm, as the child feels complicit in the abuse and thus cannot legitimise it as abusive. In addition, the lack of control over their physical arousal can create confusion and lead to a sense of betrayal by their own body.

Impact

The impact of SSA will vary from child to child and later adult depending on the age and developmental stage of the child when first abused, gender of the harmed sibling, and the sibling who has harmed, as well as the frequency and duration of the abuse, the nature of the sibling relationship, and the degree of access to social support. In addition, some children are more resilient than others and have the capacity to remain connected which can mitigate the impact, long-term effects, and therapeutic outcome, and professionals need to guard against assuming that all children experience or react to SSA in the same way. While there are many commonalities there are also many differences, and professionals need to be open to a range of reactions unique to each child and later adult.

> ### Jenna
> Jenna and her three sisters unbeknownst to each other were systemically sexually abused by their older half-brother who was often left in charge of them when their parents were away. Each of the sisters felt powerless and unable to speak out, and became highly dissociated. As children they managed to camouflage their sexual abuse and displayed no overt signs of harm. As they grew into adulthood three of the sisters developed delayed trauma reactions leading one sister to develop severe psychiatric symptoms and having to be sectioned. Another sister left the country as soon as she was able to leave home, and severed all contact with the family, while Jenna entered long-term therapy to make sense of what happened to her. The youngest sister continued to normalise the abuse, showing no outward signs of harm, and believed that her abuse had no negative impact on her.

Professionals will also need to be aware of variation in processing capacity, resilience, and access to family and social support. Very young children who are sexually abused are more likely to dissociate as they do not have the cognitive capacity to make sense of their experiences or to process them. As a result they may not be able to remember their abuse and are more likely to somatise their experiences through bodily responses that they are unable to link to the abuse experience. Older children may be more aware that it is not appropriate and extract a different meaning. They may also be more aware of the effect of disclosure on the harming sibling and the family and decide not to disclose and continue to submit, and feel more ashamed as they feel complicit in not being able to stop the sexual contact.

While the duration of the abuse increases the risk of later mental health difficulties, it is crucial to see this within the context of other factors such as the severity of the abuse and the use of force (Ballantine, 2012) as well as availability of family support, and the effects of other ACEs. The frequency and duration of SSA will impact on the degree of trauma symptoms, with prolonged and repeated abuse leading to more pervasive symptoms, especially when the abuse straddles a number of developmental stages (Sanderson, 2004). The developmental stage when the abuse occurred will influence the capacity for understanding and making meaning of their experiences and how they react to them. Moreover, young children will think and act differently, and differ in their emotional functioning than older children, and pre-verbal children who lack language and are too terrified to speak will not be able to express what has happened to them or how they feel and will be at risk of developing selective mutism or alexithymia. As a result they may only be able to communicate what is happening in a non-verbal way through their behaviour or through images. This was Marianne's experience during her sexual abuse by her violent older sister which rendered her mute for periods of time in her childhood. When she eventually started to speak she could not express her emotions and could only communicate what she felt through images and metaphors, even as an adult in therapy.

Experiences that may be perceived as traumatic by an older child may not be perceived in the same way by a younger child. Thus, a young child who does not have cognitive understanding of sex and what is considered appropriate sexual behaviour may experience the sexual contact as pleasurable and comforting without recognising it as abusive, often until many years later when they first start dating, or become intimate or have sex.

> ### Marie
> Marie was sexually abused by her older brother whom she adored and looked up to. Marie felt that this had not affected her adversely until she started adult sexual relationships when she would freeze and dissociate, and go through the motions, culminating in uncontrollable crying or fits of anger and rage after each sexual encounter.

Early SSA will also have an impact on the child's self-concept, their view of the world, and their ability to regulate themselves (Van der Kolk, 2015). Some children internalise their abuse by suppressing all feelings and developing compensatory strategies such as being cheerful, smiley, and confident, while others externalise their abuse experiences. Examples of these may include excessive washing or bathing, including the use of disinfectant or bleach to erase the feeling of being dirty and filthy, or covering up their body even in the heat of summer. Alternatively some externalise their inner feelings of being filthy by refusing to wash or bathe, and hope that being smelly will repel any potential sexual advances.

Trauma Reactions

The most common trauma responses to SSA include emotional dysregulation, PTSD symptoms, dissociation (Sanderson, 2017), shame (Sanderson, 2015), and repetitive thinking and ruminations. These in turn lead to alterations in the sense of self and self-identity as they become defined by the abuse and the abuser. Children who live under constant threat have to adapt their identity and sense of self and how they relate to others, with some children becoming submissive and compliant, while others act out their abuse by displaying anger and aggression, often towards younger siblings. This can lead to a cascade of SSA within the family. A potent example of this is in larger families in which each sibling experiences sexual abuse.

Toxic Stress

The distress and stress associated with SSA while initially experienced as tolerable will transmute into chronic and toxic stress if it persists over time (Shonkoff & Bales, 2011). As the SSA is prolonged and there is no escape the stress response system stays on high alert, and resets the alarm system. This is compounded if there is no adult to act as a 'buffer' or protect the child and thereby reduce the threat response. As a result the threat system remains high alert with the child becoming hyper-vigilant to threat cues, whether external or internal. In addition, the elevated activation of the subcortical arousal system reduces cortical functioning and deactivation of the frontal lobes which impairs executive functioning, attention, concentration, thinking, and decision making as there is no 'brake' to regulate impulsive or explosive behaviour.

When in danger or a state of terror, the body's alarm system is activated to release a cascade of neuro and biochemicals such as adrenaline and the stress hormone cortisol to prepare the body for 'fight, flight, or freeze'. These reactions are activated outside of conscious awareness and are not under voluntary control. Although the fight response consists primarily of anger and aggression, it can also include more subtle fight responses such as saying no, or screaming. The flight response ranges from physically moving away, running or hiding, to withdrawing physically or psychologically by shrinking or making oneself invisible, or dissociation. While these two responses are designed to thwart the threat, they can put the child in more danger due to the size and power differential, thus making it hard for the child to fight or flee. As a result, the child is compelled to submit through the activation of the freeze response wherein he or she becomes immobile in frozen terror, which all too often is misinterpreted by the abuser as consent. Alternatively, the child may pretend to be asleep in the hope that the abuser will leave them alone.

As immobility in the freeze response prevents the biochemicals and cortisol from being discharged, they continue to circulate in the body and send signals to the brain that the threat remains. This means the alarm system stays on high alert and the body is in a permanent state of preparedness and hyper-arousal.

Alongside the cascade of biochemicals, fear and threat also activate the social engagement system and two further threat responses, 'friend' and 'faint', that are commonly seen in response to SSA. In children the initial response to danger is to seek connection to others so that they can be protected from the threat. This signalling of danger is known as the friend response and is characterised by crying or screaming in the hope of being rescued. However, when the danger is someone known to the child, and they are prevented from crying, this may manifest as negotiating, pleading or bribing, or appeasement behaviours such as smiling or laughing which represent unconscious attempts to engage with the abuser.

If the friend reaction fails, and the threat is repeated and prolonged, the faint response will be activated and the body will dissolve into a floppy state in which muscle tension is lost and both body and mind become malleable as the body yields and higher brain functioning comes 'offline'. This submissive survival mechanism ensures that the child will become utterly submissive and compliant and show no signs of protest as they bend to the will of the abuser.

In systematic and repeated trauma, the constant flood of biochemicals will, over time, change the emotional alarm system to always be on high alert and hyper-vigilant to both internal and external cues to danger. This hyper-arousal leads to hyper-sensitivity and high levels of anxiety, irritability, impulsivity, or anger as the alarm system is easily tripped at the slightest sense of perceived danger, leading the child to respond to the world in a fearful or defensive way. In contrast some children become hypo-aroused and shut down by withdrawing or dissociating.

Emotional Dysregulation

Commonly children who have experienced SSA or trauma will experience emotional dysregulation with fluctuations between feeling really frightened, angry, or sad and feeling safe without any identifiable triggers, which can lead to extreme changes in mood and equilibrium. Activation of the threat system means that subcortical activity predominates, leading to emotional dysregulation and fluctuations in emotional functioning which are difficult to regulate.

It also reduces cortical functioning such as executive functioning, memory, concentration, focused attention, thinking, planning and decision making, and inhibition of impulse control. As higher order thinking is impaired, children struggle with the regulation of cognitive process, as well as emotional and social skills, as they are unable to exert control over powerful and overwhelming emotions. As the ability to filter relevant from irrelevant information is decreased the child alarm system becomes set on high alert leading to hyper-vigilance and the perception that the world and relationships are dangerous.

Prolonged time in such states impairs cognitive processing such as memory, concentration, reasoning, and learning, as there is no 'brake' to moderate or contain emotions, which can lead to impulsivity, violent behaviour, depression, alcohol, and substance abuse in adolescence or adulthood, and stress-related diseases. In addition, reduced cognitive processing and lack of emotional support can lead to impaired reflective functioning, metacognition, and mentalisation. As the child is in a continuous state of threat, anxiety, and confusion, there is no opportunity to reflect on their experiences, making it hard to hold self and others in mind. This reduces their capacity to understand self and others in terms of feelings, needs, desires, wishes, goals, or intentional mental states. This lack of mentalisation can lead to difficulties in the child's development of self and how they are able to relate to others.

Trauma-Related Psychiatric Disorders

Some children who have experienced SSA may display a number of challenging behaviours that can lead to psychiatric diagnoses such as PTSD, C-PTSD, and DTD. In some cases their symptoms are misunderstood or misdiagnosed as oppositional defiant disorder, attention-deficit/hyper-activity disorder (ADHD), bi-polar disorder, depression, or personality disorders, rather than a trauma-related diagnosis.

Post-Traumatic Stress Disorder

The general criteria for diagnosing PTSD applies to adults and any person over the age of six years old (Cohen & Scheeringa, 2009). There is also a dissociative subtype of PTSD, which includes all the symptoms in PTSD along with core dissociative symptoms of derealisation and depersonalisation (see below) and a separate criteria for PTSD subtype in children under the age of six which is designed to be more developmentally appropriate for young children (American Psychiatric Association, 2013). According to the *Diagnostic and Statistical Manual of Mental Disorders, Fifth Edition* (DSM-5; American Psychiatric Association, 2013), PTSD can develop at any age after one year of age and can vary according to developmental stage, with younger children less likely to display fearful reactions at the time of exposure to SSA, or when re-experiencing it, and more likely to express symptoms through play. The preschool child is also less likely to display negative self-beliefs and blame, as these are dependent on the ability to verbalise cognitive constructs and complex emotional states.

While some children who have experienced SSA develop PTSD, it is important to be mindful that not all of them will. Children, like adults, are more likely to develop PTSD if they have experienced other traumatic events, or have had a number of adverse childhood experiences, due to the cumulative effect of trauma. Research has shown that the more family and social support that the child or adolescent receives through secure and safe connections with family members, teachers, peers, and professionals, the less likely they are to develop PTSD.

A child with PTSD is likely to be plagued by constant, scary thoughts and memories of a past event which they relive over and over again, along with nightmares or flashbacks. If such symptoms occur for more than one month and negatively affect the child's life or are accompanied by depression, anxiety, or suicidal thoughts, they are more likely to be diagnosed with PTSD.

Post-Traumatic Stress Disorder Subtype in Preschool Children
Characteristics of PTSD in children six or younger include recurring, spontaneous, and intrusive upsetting memories or dreams of the traumatic event. They may also experience flashbacks or dissociative responses wherein the child feels or acts as if the event were happening again, which is often expressed through play. In addition they may experience strong and long-lasting emotional distress after being reminded of the event or after encountering trauma-related cues, or they may have strong physical reactions, such as increased heart rate or sweating.

These are often accompanied by a number of avoidance symptoms or changes in mood or thoughts. Commonly they might avoid activities, places, people, or conversations that trigger or remind the child of the traumatic event. They may also display frequent negative emotional states, such as fear, sadness, or shame along with a reduced expression of positive emotions all of which can lead to social withdrawal and lack of interest in activities that used to be meaningful or fun. Changes in arousal and reactivity are another criteria in diagnosing PTSD in preschool children. These include hyper-vigilance, which consists of being on guard all the time and unable to relax, exaggerated startle response, difficulties concentrating, as well as increased irritability, angry or violent outbursts, temper tantrums, reckless behaviour, and problems with sleeping.

Complex Post-Traumatic Stress Disorder
C-PTSD is more likely to develop in cases of multiple ACEs such as substance misuse, parental discord, physical/emotional abuse, and

neglect, and if the abuse is repeated and prolonged with no opportunity to escape, and is experienced within a relational context as in SSA, and in which there is an absence of care and protection. While care and protection may be available from adults in cases of SSA, the need for silence and secrecy precludes the child from accessing this.

The diagnostic criteria for C-PTSD includes all the features of PTSD plus severe and persistent difficulties with regulating and controlling emotions, believing oneself permanently damaged or worthless, as well as feeling shameful, guilty, or a failure; and difficulties in sustaining relationships and in feeling close to others (World Health Organization, 2018). These all challenge the child's sense of safety and personal and bodily integrity, as well as creating attachment difficulties with parents, caregivers, other family members, peers, and other adults such as teachers.

Developmental Trauma Disorder
DTD, which was originally not included in the DSM-5 (American Psychiatric Association, 2013), has generated considerable research and offers a more multi-faceted diagnosis specific to children (Van der Kolk et al., 2019; Spinazzola et al., 2021). In contrast to PTSD and C-PTSD, DTD takes into account the developmental stage during which the trauma occurred, and disruptions to key developmental tasks and concomitant symptoms, which in turn influence later developmental stages. For example, forming healthy attachments in early childhood provides the basis for forming healthy interpersonal relationships with peers in middle and late childhood, and developing a sense of self-identity.

In addition, DTD specifies a broader range of symptoms leading to emotional, cognitive, somatic, behavioural, and relational changes including confusion, dissociation, depersonalisation, clingy, compliant, or oppositional behaviour, anxiety, mood swings, impulsivity, aggression, as well as difficulties sleeping, learning difficulties, and impaired relationships. These are accompanied by altered attributions such as negative self-attributions, self-blame, mistrust, and loss of expectancy of protection by others, and risk of future victimisation. Older children and adolescents may try to self-medicate their pain or confusion through addictive behaviours involving the use of alcohol, drugs or food, gambling, sexual compulsions, or self-harm as a way to regulate unbearable emotional turmoil, or to come out of emotional shut down and dissociation.

Signs of SSA in Children and Young People

Alongside the clinical criteria to meet a diagnosis of PTSD, C-PTSD, and DTD, there are a number of symptoms in children and young people that are warning signs that they are experiencing some form of sexual trauma, including SSA. While Table 5.2 below lists the most common ones it is by no means exhaustive and there may be additional behaviours that are not listed. Practitioners and parents need to be aware that these symptoms could be due to other types of trauma or ACEs, and view these within the context of other concerns alongside SSA.

Table 5.2 Signs of sibling sexual abuse

Age 0-5	Age 5-12	Age 12-18
Become insecure and cling in fearful way	Hyper-vigilant – nervous, jittery, or alert and watchful	Emotional dysregulation – sudden outbursts of anger, irritability
Show fear of particular sibling	Detached, dissociative, daydreaming, numb, shut down, losing touch with reality	Hyper-aroused – hyper-vigilant, on edge
Cry hysterically when clothes removed, or nappy changed – not easily soothed	Negative thoughts – unlovable, filthy, bad, no good	Shut down, detached, dissociated
Recurring unexplained illnesses or genital infections – soreness or bleeding in throat, anal, or genital area	Flashbacks – images, sounds, smells, feelings	Social anxiety – withdrawn, isolated
	Overly compliant	Chronically depressed
	Difficulty concentrating or focusing at school – impaired school performance, school refusal	Negative thoughts and emotions
Regress to much younger behaviour	Changes in behaviour – aggressive, withdrawn, wary, watchful	Avoiding things they used to enjoy
Stare blankly – unhappy, confused, sad, worried	Avoids previously liked activities	Suicidal ideation and attempts
Frozen watchfulness	Reluctant to undress – gym, swimming	Unexplained pregnancies
Loss of appetite and weight loss	Avoid people or places where abuse is happening	Memory loss
Nightmares or night terrors	Eating disorders	Inappropriately sexual with others – adults, children, younger siblings
	Excessive gaming or social media use	Not able to go out with friends or invite them home

Bedwetting or soiling	Act in sexually inappropriate way – children, others	Trouble sleeping – recurring nightmares, insomnia
Shut down	Draw sexually explicit pictures depicting acts of abuse	Chronic ailments – stomach, headaches, sore throats
Fear of being separated from parent or caregiver	Urinary infections – bleeding or soreness in genital, anal area	Inability to concentrate or focus – changes in academic attainment
Fear response around harming sibling	Chronic ailments – stomach pains, headaches, sore or bleeding throat	Eating disorders
Re-enactment of the abuse through play – obsessive sexually inappropriate behaviour with dolls or other children	Regress to younger behaviour	Self-harm – self-mutilation
	Running away from home	Excessive gaming or social media use
	Lying, stealing, cheating in hopes of being caught	Excessive use of alcohol or drugs to self-medicate
	Hints about secrets	Impulsivity – risky sexual behaviour
Fear of touch or affection	Difficulty sleeping – insomnia or nightmares	Aggressive or violent – pyromania
Acting out sexually	Negative self-beliefs and self-blame, guilt, shame	Fear of intimacy, relationships, and sex
	Pseudo-maturity	
	Uncomfortable with closeness	Excessive use of pornography – violent, or child abuse images
	Depressed	
	Worrying – dying at a young age, suicidal ideation	
	Pyromania	Act out sexually – HSB, sexual violence
	Excessive use of pornography	
	Re-enacting the abuse – HSB, act out sexually	

As the impact of SSA is complex and affects children on a number of dimensions it is important that parents, family members, and professionals have greater awareness and understanding of the sexually abused child. The following chapter will examine how dissociation and shame impact on the child and their sense of self, and how this links to intrusive thoughts, ruminations, and negative self-beliefs. Equipped with this parents and professionals will be more able to understand the sexually abused child and respond more appropriately.

Further Reading

Caffaro, J. (2020). Sibling abuse of other children. In R. Geffner, V. Vieth, V. Vaughan-Eden, A. Rosenbaum, L. Hamberger, & J. White (eds), *Handbook of Interpersonal Violence across the Lifespan*. Springer.

Caffaro, J.V., & Conn-Caffaro, A. (1998). *Sibling abuse trauma: Assessment and intervention strategies for children, families and adults*. Routledge.

McCartan, K., Anning, A., & Qureshi, E. (2021). *The impact of sibling sexual abuse on adults who were harmed as children*. UWE, Bristol Research Report.

Sanderson, C. (2006). *Counselling adult survivors of child sexual abuse* (3rd edn). Jessica Kingsley Publishers.

Sanderson, C. (2013). *Counselling skills for working with trauma*. Jessica Kingsley Publishers.

Sanderson, C. (2015). *Counselling skills for working with shame*. Jessica Kingsley Publishers.

Sanderson, C. (2022). *The warrior within: A One in Four handbook to aid recovery for survivors of childhood sexual abuse and violence* (4th edn). One in Four.

Yates, P., & Allardyce, S. (2021). *Sibling sexual abuse: Knowledge and practice*. Centre of Expertise on Child Sexual Abuse.

CHAPTER 6

Understanding the Sexually Abused Child

As the impact of SSA is complex and affects children on a number of dimensions it is important that parents, family members, and professionals have greater awareness and understanding of the sexually abused child. The following chapter will examine how dissociation and shame impact on the child and their sense of self, and how this links to intrusive thoughts, ruminations, and negative self-beliefs. Equipped with this, parents and professionals will be more able to understand the sexually abused child and respond more appropriately.

Dissociation in Children
Children commonly dissociate during frightening or overwhelming experiences, or when they feel helpless, confused, or unable to escape a dangerous situation as it allows them to momentarily block out thoughts, feelings, or memories about the traumatic experience (Putnam, 1993). They typically feel as if in a dream or somewhere else in the room watching what is happening as they block off thoughts, feelings, sensations, or memories about the traumatic experience. This is especially in the case of very young children who are more likely to dissociate as they do not have the cognitive capacity to understand or process what has happened to them. With repeated trauma and over time dissociation can become a default setting even in non-traumatic situations as a way of compartmentalising all feelings and thoughts, and lead to sensitised dissociative symptoms (Perry, 2019). As dissociation becomes the default setting, it prevents the child from being fully present in their everyday lives which can negatively impact the development of a cohesive and integrated sense of self and identity as well as compromise their hold on reality.

Most children are not aware that they dissociate as they believe it is normal and cannot put what is happening to them into words. This makes it hard for adults and professionals to fully understand the range of dissociative behaviours leading to misunderstanding and mislabelling. Children are often viewed as 'zoned out', inattentive and unfocused, forgetful, slow or dozy, daydreamers, liars, or defiant in not responding when challenged. Their at-times confusing or challenging behaviours can be misdiagnosed as oppositional defiant disorder or ADHD. To help parents and professionals to identify whether the child is dissociative they can use the Child Dissociative Checklist in children ages 6–12 years, or check the common dissociative symptoms found in Box 6.1.

A degree of dissociation is normal in life, such as mild disconnection from conscious awareness when 'on autopilot', daydreaming, or immersed in reading a book or watching a film or box set. Dissociation is also a natural, adaptive way for the mind and body to protect against overwhelming emotions and experiences by anesthetising physical and psychogenic pain in order to survive adverse experiences until safety can be restored. Trauma-induced dissociation is typically more severe as the mind and body are separated, and memories and unbearable feelings and experiences are placed into different compartments (Lanius et al., 2020).

It can be challenging to detect dissociation in children because it is happening in the child's mind and the symptoms and behaviours are misunderstood by parents and professionals and viewed as shyness, daydreaming or spacing out or poor concentration, and lack of attention or focus (Perry, 2019). As dissociation in children is poorly understood they are often misdiagnosed with attention and concentration problems, learning difficulties, ADHD or conduct disorders such as oppositional defiant disorder, or psychoses (Perry, 2019). It is essential that dissociation in children who have experienced SSA is assessed and that dissociative symptoms are identified so that they are provided with the appropriate therapeutic intervention.

According to Perry (2019) the first step in the dissociation continuum is for children to make themselves invisible by blending in and staying under the radar. This protects them from being seen and reduces the risk of being abused. As they avoid others and retreat into themselves and make themselves small they are often viewed as shy, quiet, or slow, and overly compliant and robotic.

As dissociation separates the mind from the body, which impairs integration of experiences and feelings in conscious awareness, it hijacks their emotional and cognitive development. This gives rise to a range of symptoms such as amnesia and memory lapses, trance-like states and slowed down responses, rapid shifts in mood and behaviour, confusing shifts in access to knowledge, memory, and skills, disturbances in sense of self, auditory and visual hallucinations, and imaginary companions.

As they emotionally shut down they become disconnected, and experience a deep sense of emptiness, numbness, or deadness, which can make them seem unreachable. They also tend to experience their surroundings as unreal, as though they are in a dream or fog, and feel disconnected from their body or as if their body belongs to someone else. They may have out-of-body experiences, such as looking down on themselves from above, or feel as though they are floating away or dissolving into a void, or that they are a robot, or a puppet being controlled by a puppet master, and as if other people around them are not real. As they become increasingly disconnected from their body they become out of contact with their emotions, bodily sensations, and somatic states, leading to a lack of self-awareness, and concomitant lack of control over their body or behaviour.

With repeated trauma, dissociation can become a way of being as thoughts, emotions, sensations, and memories are compartmentalised, and banished from conscious awareness. This separation can lead to the fragmentation of experiences and the inability to create a coherent narrative of the abuse, or make sense of what has happened and is happening to them. In essence, trauma-related dissociation can become chronic and result in a disconnection with reality, a disconnection in interpersonal relationships, a disconnection in behaviours, and a disconnection in the self (Schimmenti & Caretti, 2016). In addition, it impairs cognitive functioning such as attention, concentration, memory, learning, and the acquisition of alternative coping skills.

In attempting to blunt the impact of trauma and ongoing threat, the child enters a state of numbness in which they are unable to feel or experience anything. Over time, dissociation can become a default setting wherein the child is so disconnected from sensations and feelings that they no longer inhabit their body and begin to live in their own world, or alternative reality. This can lead to sensitised dissociative symptoms such as perceptual disturbances in time or size, and physical symptoms such as fainting, gastrointestinal problems, and recurring unexplained illness (Perry, 2019). Dissociation can lead to poor concentration and lack of focus and attention as the child is absorbed in their inner traumatised world. This can lead to impaired processing of information and learning. Conversely, some children find comfort in immersing themselves into accumulating knowledge and learning in order to distract themselves from the abuse, and compensate for the harm they have experienced through achievement and academic success. This can make them feel less powerless and feel valued for their knowledge and skills.

Persistent dissociation can lead to depersonalisation in which a child's sense of self and identity becomes confused, and in which they are unsure about who they are, and experience their body as unreal, changing, or dissolving. They can also become detached from their body and have out-of-body experiences, or feel as though they are watching themselves in a dream or film rather than actually experiencing what is happening to them. This is often experienced as feeling dead inside or like a robot, and as if their body has been hijacked or dissolved.

Severe dissociation can also lead to derealisation in which the world seems unreal, where the familiar is unfamiliar, where friends become unreal or turn into robots and objects appear to change in shape, size, or colour, and time speeds up or slows down. The overall experience is saturated with vague and dreamlike states which are typically described as being in a haze or fog.

A more complex and bewildering type of dissociation is structural dissociation wherein a division in the personality or identity occurs which prevents the development of a cohesive sense of self, or fragments any acquired cohesive self-structure (Van der Hart et al., 2006). This can result in the formation of separate and discrete self-states, which are not consciously accessible. This can range from a simple division between a seemingly Apparently Normal Personality which is highly functional in everyday life, and an Emotional Personality which is immersed in trauma and trauma reactions, to extremely complex divisions of the personality into multiple identities as seen in dissociative identity disorder (Van der Hart et al., 2006). Structural dissociation disrupts the fluidity and flexibility of self-states, preventing the child from identifying with 'I' statements as they do not have a unitary or cohesive sense of self, due to disowned self-states and aspects of the self. The younger the child at the time of the SSA the greater the impact of structural dissociation and the development of multiple parts, while older children who have acquired a more cohesive sense of self will experience less fragmentation primarily (Van der Hart et al., 2006).

Children with trauma-generated structural dissociation often present as chaotic as they switch between alternate self-states which is confusing for adults and professionals as they are unable to make sense of their responses and behaviours (Van der Hart et al., 2006), and are often misdiagnosed with oppositional disorders or conduct disorder as children, while adolescents and adults are mislabelled with personality disorders, such as borderline personality disorder (emotional unstable personality disorder), narcissistic personality disorder, or antisocial personality disorder.

In both structural dissociation and dissociative identity disorder the mind 'splits off' emotions, physical sensations, and aspects of self-experience which can be 'held' through the formation of separate parts or identities (International Society for the Study of Trauma and Dissociation, 2011), such as the functioning part, the traumatised part, the hurt or angry child part. While having multiple dissociative parts can appear confusing to others, the child may not be aware of these parts. Moreover, these separate parts can be helpful to the child as each serves a purpose in the child's survival. For example a fighting part helps the child to fight for survival, while an angry part can hold the anger that is too dangerous to express, or the smiley, bright, and bubbly part ensures that the secret is kept, and the compliant and submissive part preserves the attachment and protects the child from further punishment or shame, while the sad part holds the sadness so the child can retain hope and function in everyday life.

Common dissociative symptoms include loss of time for minutes, hours, or sometimes days, as well as time distortions. This can lead to gaps in memory as well as total memory loss, both for past and recent events or conversations, as well as loss of skills and personal information about themselves. It is these symptoms that are often behind mood swings, personality shifts, forgetfulness, dreamlike states, inattention, or memory loss for periods of time. These can all be confusing and frightening for the child especially if they can't remember who they are, where they were, or what they were doing. In addition, dissociation often underpins other mental health problems such as depression, bi-polar disorder, anxiety disorders, personality disorders, self-harm, obsessive compulsive disorder (OCD), sleep disturbances such as nightmares, night terrors, night-time flashbacks or panic attacks and parasomnias such as sleep walking, and the range of symptoms seen in PTSD, C-PTSD, and DTD.

It is important to acknowledge that dissociation occurs suddenly outside of conscious awareness and outside of voluntary control. Knowing this can reduce the sense of shame and self-blame that many people feel and help them to understand their reactions within the context of trauma (Sanderson, 2017, 2022).

> Box 6.1 Common dissociative symptoms in children (adapted from Choi et al., 2018)
>
> - Amnesia for important or traumatic events known to have occurred
> - Dazed or trance-like states – daydreaming, blanking out, spaciness, zoned out, avoidance of eye contact
> - Glazed look in the eyes, rolling or fluttering of the eyes indicating switching from the here and now to a dissociative state. May move eyes from side to side, or up and down, rub their eyes or blink rapidly as though they are trying to blink their way out of the dissociated state, shake head excessively, rub their face or touch parts of their body in order to check if it, and they, are still there
> - Confusion and disorientation
> - Slower, less efficient processing including slowed down bodily movement, over contained, immobile, and frozen watchfulness. Slow to finish tasks such as getting dressed or getting ready to go out
> - Memory lapses for seconds, minutes, or hours at a time. Can include things they have said or done, including challenging behaviour or misdemeanours which they have no memory of and thus deny
> - Forgetfulness of information, facts, or skills they have learned such as reading, handwriting, or riding a bike – can fluctuate from day to day
> - Suddenly can't speak and stop mid-sentence as they have lost words, or can't remember what was said
> - Alterations in awareness of time, space, and sense of self. Confusion and disorientation around time of day, where they are, or who they are. Perceptual distortions in time, size, colour, and shapes

- Mercurial mood shifts without any obvious triggers wherein they oscillate between being calm or feeling safe, and then frightened, sacred, angry, or sad
- Volatile changes in behaviour or appearance without any obvious triggers such as changes in dress, hairstyle, tone and rhythm of voice, use of language, muscle tone, or handwriting
- Unable to do tasks and follow instructions, often due to not being able to 'hear', understand, or process what is required of them
- Overly compliant and submissive or avoidant and defiant
- Distracted by internal voices or conversations – auditory and visual hallucinations
- Repeatedly referring to themselves in the third person, saying 'we' or 'they' as if they have multiple parts or identities, behaving and speaking in different voices
- Vivid imaginary companion(s) that control the child's behaviour
- Sudden age regression – in which they look, sound, and behave much younger than they are
- Self-injurious behaviour in order to calm themselves or bring them out of a dissociate state, such as slapping themselves or head bashing to wake themselves up, or to calm and soothe themselves. This can become a form of emotional self-regulation which can become addictive and compulsive. The more dissociative the child is the greater the need for intense stimulation to penetrate dissociative states such as cutting, picking, scratching, masturbating until they bleed
- Somatisation and recurring physical illnesses without medical explanation – tummy aches, headaches, light headedness, fainting

Dissociation in Adolescents

Adolescents who have a diagnosis of dissociation PTSD subtype have been found to have more trauma experiences as well as more severe PTSD and problems with behaviour. Alongside this, they tend to experience more daydreaming and dissociative amnesia, including memory problems, forgetting things, and blocking out thoughts when compared to adults with that diagnosis (Choi et al., 2018).

It is crucial that parents and professionals can identify the signs of dissociation so they can fully understand what is happening to the child rather than mislabelling their symptoms. In addition, it is helpful to recognise that dissociation can be beneficial as it keeps them safe when they are overwhelmed and gives them a temporary reprieve from unbearable feelings. Dissociation can be a healthy adaptive mechanism which can aid creativity and help children to self-regulate and survive trauma (Perry, 2019). In recognising that dissociative symptoms are a form of self-regulation, parents and professionals can introduce other forms of healthy self-regulation to ground themselves and reduce the need to dissociate and remain connected to themselves and the present.

Impact on Attachment
Trauma and SSA hijacks the attachment system making it extremely hard to trust others or get close to them as they have learnt that relationships are a source of danger and confusion rather than a source of comfort. In addition, the fear that closeness can be sexualised necessitates keeping people at bay either by avoiding them, or being aggressive or hostile. This creates a paradox in which the child yearns for closeness and yet is compelled to avoid it. As a result, children make themselves invisible in relationships to avoid getting hurt.

As the attachment system becomes activated the child can become either fearfully dependent and clingy, or, if deactivated, avoid getting close to others. Either way, they become hyper-vigilant in monitoring others' moods and adjust their mood accordingly, and attempt to 'mind read' others in order to brace themselves for any potential danger or harm. As they become more sensitised to others' needs they become more concerned about pleasing others, and take responsibility for their emotional well-being and compulsively put their needs first to try to make them feel better. This is often the case in SSA, where the harmed sibling goes to great lengths to protect the harming sibling as they do not want them to get in trouble or be responsible for causing conflict in the family. This was palpable in Sonia's case who felt sorry for her brother as he was always in trouble and she wanted to protect him from getting into more trouble by not disclosing that he was regularly coming into her room at night and forcing her to perform oral sex on him.

This can impact on their attachment style not just in relation to their siblings, but also towards their parents, peers, and relationships in adulthood. While some children and later adults will have little or no contact with the sibling who has harmed them, others will preserve and continue to sustain their relationship throughout their adult life (Finkelhor et al., 1989; Myers, et al., 2002; Courtois & Ford, 2012; Stroebel et al., 2013; Caffaro and Conn-Caffaro, 2014).

Traumatised and abused children tend to develop insecure attachment styles such as anxious-avoidant attachment, anxious-preoccupied attachment, or disorganised attachment. Children with anxious-avoidant attachment style are fiercely independent, and feel anxious when someone gets too close, leading them to avoid relationships. As it is important for them to feel self-sufficient they find it hard to reach out or seek help, and thus avoid showing distress. This leads to a fear of making friends or developing close relationships which can persist into adulthood, which prevents them from learning and building relationship skills, and ultimately leads to isolation and loneliness as they become locked in a psychological prison. In contrast the children with an anxious-preoccupied attachment style seek constant reassurance and exaggerate distress to elicit a caring response. They tend to be overly dependent on others and clingy as they require constant validation and reassurance, and panic and worry when on their own.

The most common attachment style associated with children who have been sexually abused is the disorganised attachment style in which the harming sibling can be both a source of comfort and harm. This unpredictability can be confusing and exhausting as the child wants to be close to the sibling and yet needs to avoid them and push them away. As a result, the child may tolerate behaviours that are confusing or harmful as they are not sure how to set boundaries and fear the consequences of asserting themselves and saying 'no' (Sanderson, 2022). As a result they may form a trauma bond with the harming sibling which is extremely hard to break. Trauma bonds tend to develop in relationships where there is a power imbalance and the person with power oscillates between caring for and harming the child. Children with a disorganised attachment style differ from those with an avoidant attachment style in that they want to be close but are terrified of getting hurt so need to withdraw, and will oscillate between approach and avoid behaviours, which can be confusing to those around them as they seek closeness and then push the person away.

Trust

Due to the betrayal of trust in SSA many children become fearful of others, which impairs their capacity to trust, leading to avoidance and withdrawal from others, isolation, and loneliness. In addition, the withdrawal prevents them from forming friendships and learning relationship skills. In addition, the need for predictability, certainty, and sense of control makes it difficult to be responsive to care and affection. While the child yearns to be loved and cared for, they are all too often terrified or suspicious of this, as love and care are associated with confusion and hurt. Many children struggle to accept being loved or cared for as they cannot accept let alone like themselves, and find it hard to believe that others might like or care for them.

Some children either trust too much in order to preserve the relationship, or mistrust not just the harming sibling but other family members, including the primary caregivers. They will typically test others to see whether they can be trusted, which can lead to challenging behaviours as they push others' limits of patience and tolerance. Children who override their fear by becoming overly trusting typically become overly compliant and submissive, and compulsively put other people's needs first, or help others as this enables them to feel more in control. In contrast, children whose attachment system is deactivated find it hard to connect to or trust others, and avoid closeness at all costs. This tends to manifest as excessive self-sufficiency, self-reliance, and independence. This pseudo-independence is rooted in the belief that 'I'm on my own', 'I cannot trust or rely on others', and 'it is shameful to ask for help', which compounds their sense of isolation and lack of belongingness. Children can also find it hard to trust themselves, which can lead to self-doubt and a chronic lack of self-agency as they fear failure or that they will make poor choices that might harm or endanger them.

Shame and Self-Blame

Another reason to push others away is to reduce any further exposure to shame (see Box 6.2). Children who have experienced sexual abuse are particularly vulnerable to developing chronic or toxic shame (Sanderson, 2022). Sexual abuse invariably also engenders self-blame, leaving the child feeling dirty, worthless, unlovable, and inadequate. The corrosive nature of shame leaves an indelible stain on the child's sense of self-worth and self-esteem, alongside overwhelming feelings of self-loathing and self-disgust, which can only be quelled by pushing them out of conscious awareness to disavow them.

The shame associated with SSA is an interplay between the shame felt at the time of the abuse and the sense of shame in the present, especially should it be exposed. Shame during the abuse is commonly due to the nature of the sexual acts, having to submit to them and not being able to defend against them. This is intensified if the child feels shame for approaching the harming sibling, or is sexually aroused or had an erection or orgasm during the sexual encounter. It is crucial to convey to the child that this does not mean they wanted to be sexually abused or are responsible for the SSA, and see this as a survival strategy. In addition, children may approach the harming sibling in order to have a semblance of control and predictability over the abuse which enables the child to armour themselves in preparation for the sexual contact and help them feel less vulnerable. Children who were aroused or enjoyed the sexual contact may seek out the sibling to repeat the sexual activity not to be abused but to re-experience the 'nice' feelings. This is a normal response in young children who do not experience SSA as abuse and seek to repeat pleasurable feelings. Parents and professionals must not judge this or make the child feel complicit.

Shame is also compounded if the child depends on the harming sibling, as they will find it hard to blame those that they depend on for fear of the consequences. They tend to blame themselves by taking on the responsibility for the abuse in order to retain a positive image of the harming sibling. This self-blame is often heightened if the harming sibling tells the child it is their fault for being seductive, or initiating the sexual contact. With the abuser not taking any responsibility for the abuse, the child has no choice but to blame themselves, and they are not able to legitimise it as abuse.

It is worth noting that self-blame can have psychological benefits such as suppressing anger and rage, thereby permitting the child to view the harming sibling as kind, loving, and caring rather than abusive. However, by taking on the responsibility for the abuse and blame itself, the child cannot legitimise the sexual contact as abusive. Self-blame also allows for a sense of control in which the child can believe that 'If only I hadn't done this…then that wouldn't have happened', which enables them to feel more in control in the face of potential abuse in the future, and hold on to the belief that others do not necessarily mean them harm.

In contrast to guilt, which focuses on actual transgressions, shame can be felt even if there has been no wrongdoing, or when it is being deflected or projected. As shame is more covert and diffuse the child is more likely to say they feel 'bad' or guilty rather than state that they feel ashamed. In shame negative evaluations are focused on the self rather than a specific behaviour or act. Thus, the whole of the self feels inferior, defective, or degraded, leading to a deep sense of self-loathing, self-contempt, and self-hatred (Sanderson, 2022). The child sees themselves as 'bad' with no possibility of reparation or atonement. The emphasis is on the rejection of the self or core identity for which there is no reparation other than to avoid exposure or by becoming invisible (Lewis, 1971; Tangney & Dearing, 2002; Sanderson, 2013).

The violation of sexual boundaries and lack of mastery over the body breeds shame and it is ubiquitous in sexual violence and SSA, especially if there is confusion around sexual excitation and pleasure during SSA. Children who were aroused during their abuse or had an erection or orgasm often feel complicit in their abuse thus intensifying their sense of shame and self-blame. Shame is also exacerbated when the child seeks out the harming sibling for affection and attention, or is not able to stop the abuse. Furthermore, the shamelessness of the harming sibling in committing the SSA is absorbed by the child, which means they not only feel their own shame but internalise the shame that is projected onto them. Finally, the lack of control that the child has over their body is a further source of shame as this prevents the child from developing mastery over their body and compromises their sense of self-agency.

As the shame in SSA is often unidentified and unaddressed, it metastasises into chronic shame leading to low self-esteem, never feeling good enough, unlovable, self-loathing, and unresolved anger. This can lead to 'shame proneness' in which the child is highly sensitised to shame cues and constant anticipation that they will be shamed by others. In order to mitigate this, and remain in control of their shame, they may perpetuate shame by shaming themselves through ruminations, mental compulsions, negative self-beliefs and self-talk, or shameless behaviour so that no-one can shame them as much as they shame themselves (Sanderson, 2015). This can give rise to acting out, hurting others, or lack of empathy and compassion for others. Alternatively they may render themselves invisible by erasing themselves and becoming self-sacrificing, feeling responsible for others, and repudiating their needs so they can focus on others to gain approval and feel 'good' rather than ashamed.

This can ultimately make them more vulnerable to not being able to set boundaries and at risk of being manipulated and exploited, or enticed into toxic relationships.

The focus of shame tends to coalesce around the body and the body in action, sense of self, feeling a failure and defective, lack of relational worth and lovability. In addition they may feel secondary shame for feeling ashamed, being dependent, vulnerable, and not defending themselves, as well as vicarious shame by introjecting the shame that belongs to others, including the harming sibling. The child becomes drenched in shame, which reinforces the need to conceal, hide, and withdraw from others to avoid exposure. This can become so paralysing that the child makes themselves smaller and smaller to blend in and stay under the radar, inhibiting spontaneity and curiosity, and slowing down movement and interaction with others. While this is often perceived as shyness or social anxiety it is likely to be trauma induced, reflecting the interplay of shame and dissociation (Sanderson, 2015).

As the experience of shame is so unbearable, the child needs to find ways to defend against it (Lewis, 1971) through the adoption of a number of masks to cover up the felt sense of shame. Nathanson (1992) proposes four distinct strategies that are used to manage or ward off shame: withdrawal, attacks on the self, avoidance, or attacking others. The primary strategy is withdrawal, by avoiding the gaze of others and any further shame. In withdrawal the child tries to become invisible by shying away from others or becoming submissive and compliant. Children who withdraw from others are often not seen to have a problem as they tend to present as model children who are eager to please, albeit somewhat shy and modest. Physically they often conceal themselves by avoiding eye contact or hiding their body by covering it up, especially when having to change for PE or swimming. These children are often inhibited in their body movements and appear rigid with little or no spontaneity. As they feel they have no control over their body, they fear bodily actions and actively avoid any type of physical performance, dance, sport, or physical exercise. In addition, they fear talking or speaking out loud in case they inadvertently reveal their shame or abuse, leading them to isolate themselves from others by avoiding closeness and friendships.

In contrast, some children engage in self-attacking strategies such as pervasive and degrading self-criticism in which they blame themselves for everything. This gives rise to negative core beliefs, negative self-thoughts, and negative self-talk, which feed a persecutory inner critic who constantly denigrates the child. This can sometimes manifest as self-deprecating humour or self-effacement that can be misconstrued as modesty or humility, which belies the depth of shame the child is feeling. Attacking the self can also lead to self-harming behaviours including self-mutilation. Children who attack the self are also more likely to suffer from suicidal ideation and a range of depressive symptoms. A danger is that as the shame is buried and not processed it can build up and emerge in explosive anger and attacks on others (Sanderson, 2015).

Alongside withdrawal, some children bypass the experience of shame through avoidance in which they attempt to deny or blank out the shame through dissociation or numbing. This is commonly achieved through a range of self-medicating behaviours to numb feelings and alter mood. In young children this may manifest as ritualised self-soothing behaviours such as thumb sucking, or rhythmic stroking of certain parts of the body including the genitals to self-regulate. In adolescents it is more likely through the use of drugs and alcohol, comfort eating, or risky behaviour in which thrill seeking distracts them from the unbearable feelings of shame. A further cover for shame is the use of compensatory strategies such as hubristic or excessive pride, self-aggrandisement, grandiosity, over self-confidence, arrogance, perfectionism, and narcissism (Nathanson, 1992; Sanderson, 2015).

Children who use the strategy of attacking others are often consumed with humiliated fury which they externalise by attacking others in the hope of expunging their own shame by projecting it onto others. Such children often present as angry, defensive, critical, hostile, and violent towards others. They typically lack empathy for others which allows them to engage in shameless acts of violence or aggression, such as bullying or HSB, in their quest to triumph over their own shame proneness (Sanderson, 2015).

Box 6.2 Shame

- Excessive self-consciousness
- Concealment of body, emotions, needs
- Shame proneness – and heightened sensitivity to shame
- Low self-esteem – self-loathing and lack of healthy self-love
- Loss of belief and trust in themselves

- Belief they are a failure
- Lack of motivation – to succeed or to do anything, don't have goals, and only do things to distract from how they feel
- Emptiness or deep chasm, or void
- Anxiety-based shyness – social anxiety
- Poor social skills
- Negative self-talk
- Withdrawal
- Avoidance of feelings, thoughts, behaviour
- Compensatory strategies such as adopting opposite feelings, thoughts, and behaviours, excessive pride, grandiosity, narcissism, grandiose fantasies to compensate for sense of worthlessness
- Perfectionism to compensate for feeling inadequate and useless
- False self – overly confident to hide feeling inferior, overly smiley to hide the hurt, overly competitive, struggle to cope with not winning
- Lack of empathy and compassion for self and others – inconsiderate to others
- Vulnerable to being manipulated or succumbing to peer pressure
- Conflicted relationship to self and others – difficulties in their relationships with parents, siblings, teachers, friends, and relatives
- Poor self-care
- Self-harm
- Suicidality
- Aggression, violence, humiliation, or shaming others to deflect shame

Negative Core Beliefs and Self-Thoughts

The felt sense of shame impacts on the child's perception of self and their self-identity. This is seen in feelings of unlovability, self-loathing, and self-disgust, that they are so flawed that others will be repulsed by them and that they have no right to exist (Sanderson, 2015, 2022). This negative view of the self is often supported by negative core beliefs about the self and negative self-thoughts which lead to ruminations, negative self-talk, and excoriating self-criticism. These tend to feed a persecutory internal critic, and erode self-esteem and self-confidence.

Typically, negative beliefs and accompanying self-talk underpin automatic thoughts that are triggered outside of conscious awareness, and consist of negative thoughts or images which can arise instantaneously and the child feels they have no control over. While initially brief they can become habitual and develop into relentless obsessive thoughts and ruminations (see Box 6.3).

Negative core beliefs commonly consist of negative thoughts about the self, others, the world, and the future. Sometimes these are so habitual that they become automatic and occur outside of conscious awareness and yet infect the developing self-identity. While these can be the internalisation of how the child has been defined by others, including the harming sibling, they can also be as a result of shame and self-blame. These negative self-beliefs are reflected in the child's inner critical voice which constantly undermines the child's feelings, thoughts, and behaviour by stripping away any vestiges of self-esteem.

Box 6.3 Common negative core beliefs

- I am unlovable
- I am filthy, dirty, and disgusting
- I am to blame
- I am worthless
- I don't matter
- I am not good enough
- Everything is my fault
- I can't do anything right
- I don't deserve good things
- I am a bad child or person
- I deserve to be treated the way others treat me
- My needs and feelings are not important
- Nobody likes me
- I can't be myself around others
- I have to hide my true emotions and thoughts

- People are dangerous and can't be trusted
- The world is not safe

Negative self-beliefs can metastasise into endless rumination and mental compulsions, especially around transgressive or repugnant thoughts about the self. Some children ruminate about causing harm to others, or that they have committed a terrible act (Veale et al., 2009). These mental compulsions can occur spontaneously and are extremely hard to control, or extinguish, as they are repeatedly replayed in the child's head. This can be exhausting and time consuming, making it hard for the child to engage in other activities, or live life fully. As they are plagued by these ruminations the child struggles to focus and concentrate, which impairs the processing of information. To neutralise negative self-beliefs and thoughts the child may impose unrealistic expectations on themselves and develop perfectionist traits through 'should' statements of how they should or ought to be or behave. As these expectations are invariably unrealistic and virtually impossible to achieve the child is destined to fail, which generates more shame and self-criticism, and fuels low self-esteem. Negative core beliefs about the self and self-criticism have a significant impact on the child's sense of self and identity.

Impact on Sense of Self

Living under prolonged threat and confusion can result in enduring personality changes (Herman, 1992) as the child needs to adapt to and accommodate the abuse and the needs and desires of others. This is exacerbated in cases of complex trauma and trauma-induced dissociation (see above in this chapter) wherein the disconnection in the self results in different components or parts of the self and individual states becoming divided, resulting in discordant and incoherent responses to the same stimuli (Schimmenti & Caretti, 2016).

This disorganisation of the self and attempts to cover up the lack of integration can promote the development of a 'false self' to conceal and suppress feelings of anger, hurt, or sadness, or weakness and vulnerability. In order for the child to survive they may develop compensatory personality traits to cover up the abuse and felt sense of shame by developing a façade of invulnerability to conceal vulnerability, a sense of omnipotence to counteract feelings of helplessness and powerlessness, grandiosity to mask a sense of inadequacy, excessive confidence to cover up their sense of failure, and excessive cheerfulness to mask oceanic sadness and hurt. A false self may also emerge as a result of being defined by others, especially the harming sibling who in defining the sibling they are harming, imposes and identity on them, which the harmed sibling introjects and subsequently overrides any previously acquired sense of self (Mollon, 2000), which is then introjected, obliterating any previously acquired sense of self.

If the SSA occurs at a very young age before the child has had the opportunity to organise mental states and develop a cohesive sense of self, the child will have difficulty organising individual self-states and their respective realities into a cohesive overarching cognitive and experiential state that is felt as 'me'. In the absence of a unified sense of self, the child will remain fragmented with multiple states of self, or parts which are experienced as separate ego states or identities.

The sense of self can also be hijacked in children who have developed a cohesive sense of self, wherein the self becomes fragmented as the child's integration of psychological functioning is compromised through trauma-induced dissociation. This results in a re-organisation of self-states which are organised around fear states and anxiety and give rise to conceptions of the self. Howell (2011, 2013) proposes that the three primary conceptions are 'good me' which is organised around affects and behaviours that have been met with approval; 'bad me' which derives from behaviours that have not been accepted; and 'not me' which are aspects of the self that have been 'split off' and pushed out of conscious awareness and dissociated, or defensively excluded (Bowlby, 1973). The more pronounced the division between 'me' and 'not me' the greater the dissociative organisation of the sense of self (Howell, 2011, 2013) in which the division of experience and knowledge prevents the child from knowing all parts of the self and attaining self-state coherence. This disruption to the developmental trajectory can result in significant impairments in the child's sense of self and behaviours.

Due to the lack of a cohesive sense of self and the split off 'not me' parts, the child struggles to identify with 'I' statements and is not consciously aware when the disavowed parts surface, and is not able to recognise or remember actions, feelings, thoughts, or behaviours they have engaged in. As the 'not me' child avoids intolerable self-experiences such as the SSA and unbearable feelings, sensations, and thoughts by detaching from them, these transmute into dissociated parts such as hurt or angry child parts, shamed parts, protector parts, or persecutory parts.

In order to hold on to the 'good me' the child will become overly compliant, extremely biddable, and submissive to gain approval and feel loved and to ensure that 'good me' is consistently reinforced. As the 'good me' is a source of praise and implies that the child is well adjusted and not experiencing any negative feelings and thoughts, such children often remain under the radar and are not identified as suffering from trauma or abuse. In contrast, children who identify with the 'bad me' externalise their anger, humiliation, and shame by acting out through hostility, defiance, aggression, violence, or harming others.

Overall, children who have experienced SSA lose their sense of self and incur damage to their identity. As they have to conceal aspects of the self, or are prevented from developing a cohesive self, they often feel different to everyone else, which comprises their sense of belongingness, while increasing their alienation from self and others. In the absence of self they are forced to develop a 'false self', or multiple selves to cover up their internal pain and confusion. As a result they become too scared and ashamed to be themselves, often leading a double life in which outwardly they appear to be well adjusted while internally they are falling apart.

Without help and appropriate intervention children who experience SSA can remain invisible and under the radar, and carry the impact of the abuse into adulthood which will manifest in a range of long-term effects, explored in the next chapter. The chapter will examine delayed trauma reactions and the risk of PTSD and C-PTSD in adulthood along with the long-term effects of SSA. It will identify the trauma symptoms associated with SSA trauma, such as dissociation, emotional dysregulation, and a range of other mental health difficulties, somatisation, and compromised physical health, as well as the use of substances such as alcohol, drugs, medication, and food to numb overwhelming emotions.

Further Reading

Caffaro, J. (2020). Sibling abuse of other children. In R. Geffner, V. Vieth, V. Vaughan-Eden, A. Rosenbaum, L. Hamberger, & J. White (eds), *Handbook of Interpersonal Violence across the Lifespan*. Springer.

Caffaro, J.V., & Conn-Caffaro, A. (1998). *Sibling abuse trauma: Assessment and intervention strategies for children, families and adults*. Routledge.

McCartan, K., Anning, A., & Qureshi, E. (2021). *The impact of sibling sexual abuse on adults who were harmed as children*. UWE, Bristol Research Report.

Myers, l. J., Berliner, L., Briere, J., Hendrix, C. T., Reid, T., & Jenny, C. (2002). Treating adult survivors of severe childhood abuse and neglect: Further development of an integrative model. *JEB Myers, L. Berliner, J. Briere, CT Hendrix, T. Reid, & C. Jenny. The APSAC handbook on child maltreatment*.

Sanderson, C. (2006). *Counselling adult survivors of child sexual abuse* (3rd edn). Jessica Kingsley Publishers.

Sanderson, C. (2013). *Counselling skills for working with trauma*. Jessica Kingsley Publishers.

Sanderson, C. (2015). *Counselling skills for working with shame*. Jessica Kingsley Publishers.

Sanderson, C. (2017). *Dissociation and dissociative disorders: Advice for adults suffering with dissociation and those working with them*. One in Four.

Sanderson, C. (2022). *The warrior within: A One in Four handbook to aid recovery for survivors of childhood sexual abuse and violence* (4th edn). One in Four.

Yates, P. (2017). Sibling sexual abuse: Why don't we talk about it? *Journal of Clinical Nursing, 26*(15-16), 2482–2494.

Yates, P., & Allardyce, S. (2021). *Sibling sexual abuse: Knowledge and practice*. Centre of Expertise on Child Sexual Abuse.

Yates, P., & Allardyce, S. (2022). Abuse at the heart of the family: The challenges and complexities of sibling sexual abuse. In K. Uzieblo, W.J. Smid, & K. McCartan (eds), *Challenges in the Management of People Convicted of a Sexual Offence*. Palgrave Macmillan.

CHAPTER 7

The Long-Term Effects of Sibling Sexual Abuse on Adult Survivors

Without help and appropriate intervention children who experience SSA can remain invisible and under the radar, and carry the impact of the abuse into adulthood which will manifest in a range of long-term effects. This chapter will examine the long-term effects on survivors including trauma reactions such as emotional dysregulation, dissociation, mental health difficulties, somatisation, and compromised physical health.

The long-term effects of SSA will vary from survivor to survivor depending on the age or gender of the child when the abuse occurred, the nature, frequency, and duration of the abuse, the relationship to and gender of the sibling who has sexually harmed them, and the degree of support from the family and professionals. It is crucial not to make assumptions that all survivors of SSA will experience or react to the SSA in the same way. While there are many commonalities such as psychological and physical health problems, impaired trust, changed and diminished sense of self, shame, and relational difficulties, there are also many differences, and professionals need to be open to a range of reactions unique to each survivor rather than try to fit them into a simplified standardised formulation.

Delayed trauma reactions and the risk of PTSD and C-PTSD in adulthood are some of the long-term effects of SSA and will be considered in this chapter along with a range of symptoms such as emotional dysregulation, shame, and the use of substances such as alcohol, drugs, medication, and food to numb overwhelming emotions. In addition, the chapter will examine the impact on the attachment system and relationships, including intimacy and sexuality. Many survivors of SSA struggle with navigating family of origin relationships, including with the sibling who harmed them, and are fearful of how to protect their own children.

The most common immediate impact of SSA on the child is one of confusion, which is often accompanied by fear and shame. Many survivors report that they did not view the SSA as abuse at the time it occurred, and often believed it to be consensual and as such normalised it (Caffaro, 2017, 2020; McCartan et al., 2021; Yates & Allardyce, 2022) and did not realise that it was harmful. While they did not necessarily experience the initial HSB as trauma it would nevertheless have resulted in confusion, doubt, and uncertainty due to the secrecy in which it was conducted. Coercive or threatening SSA that is repeated and protracted activates the threat response system leading to elevated levels of fear and stress, emotional dysregulation, and a range of trauma reactions and symptoms (Sanderson, 2022).

This commonly manifests in adult survivors as 'delayed trauma' or delayed-onset PTSD or C-PTSD, and can include persistent fatigue, flashbacks, sleep disorders, nightmares, anxiety, fear, depression, and avoidance of emotions, sensations, or activities that are associated with the trauma.

Post-Traumatic Stress Disorder and Complex Post-Traumatic Stress Disorder

The primary symptoms in PTSD are intrusive, such as flashbacks, nightmares, sleep disturbances, and memories which are often accompanied by high levels of arousal and reactivity as seen in hyper-arousal, hypervigilance, exaggerated startle response, problems with concentration, or hypo-arousal and loss of awareness of present surroundings (American Psychiatric Association, 2013; World Health Organization, 2018).

As these are so distressing, survivors commonly avoid memories, thoughts, feelings, people, places, or situations associated with the traumatic experience. In addition, there are persistent overwhelming feelings such as fear, terror, anger, and shame that lead to mood swings, as well as negative thoughts and feelings about the self, others, and the world. This is often accompanied by loss of interest in significant activities, feelings of detachment or estrangement from others, and due to a sense of numbness an inability to experience feelings, including positive emotions such as pleasure, joy, or love.

It is critical that these symptoms are seen as normal responses to abnormal events, not as signs of weakness or irrationality, and this must be conveyed to the survivor. It is also important to understand just how disruptive, distracting, and disturbing these symptoms can be to a survivor's everyday life, to the performance of everyday tasks and to their physical health, as they live continually 'on edge' which is exhausting. It is these trauma symptoms that lead to self-medication, self-harm, and a range of anxiety disorders and negative self-beliefs and thoughts.

PTSD is characterised by a number of symptoms which coalesce around intrusion symptoms, avoidance, negative alterations in mood, and alterations in arousal and reactivity. Intrusion symptoms consist of persistent re-experiencing of the trauma through involuntary and intrusive memories, nightmares, dissociative reactions such as flashbacks which can range from brief episodes to complete loss of awareness, and prolonged periods of distress, often accompanied by increased heart rate and intense physiological arousal. Avoidance symptoms are characterised by avoiding trauma-related reminders such as trauma-related inner experiences (e.g. thoughts or feelings) or external reminders (e.g. people, places, activities, objects, situations, or conversations).

Negative alterations in mood and cognitions include dissociative amnesia which is characterised by an inability to recall key features of the trauma, and persistent negative beliefs and expectations about oneself, others, or the world such as 'I am bad' or 'relationships are dangerous'. This is usually accompanied by a distorted sense of self-blame and responsibility for the SSA and its consequences and concomitant persistent negative emotions such as fear, anger, shame, and the inability to experience positive feelings such as joy, happiness, or love. Survivors who have dissociative symptoms will experience depersonalisation and derealisation in which they feel alienated, detached, or estranged from self, others, and the world (see Chapter 4).

Alterations in arousal and reactivity consist of hyper-arousal and hyper-vigilance; exaggerated startle response; irritability; aggressive, self-destructive, impulsive, or reckless behaviour; as well as problems in concentration and sleep disturbance. In contrast some survivors of SSA become hypo-aroused wherein they become shut down, detached, and unreachable. These trauma reactions result in considerable emotional dysregulation which is easily triggered by external as well as internal cues associated with the abuse, leading to outbursts of rage, aggression, or violence, or withdrawal and shut down.

C-PTSD encompasses all of the symptoms seen in PTSD along with pronounced emotional dysregulation, dissociative states with periods of loss of attention and concentration, pervasive feelings of shame or guilt, negative view of self, and relationship difficulties including withdrawal from friends and family. It can also be accompanied by the somatisation of the trauma in physical symptoms such as chronic fatigue, headaches, dizziness, chest pains, stomach aches, and unexplained medical illnesses (Sanderson, 2022).

Emotional Dysregulation

Trauma reactions such as hyper- and hypo-arousal can interfere with the ability to regulate emotions. Some survivors become stuck in either of the two extremes, while others swing between the two. As the hyper-arousal escalates and the emotional intensity threatens to overwhelm, many survivors 'short circuit' by numbing emotions through alcohol, drugs, food, or sex, or dissociating. Alternatively some resort to self-harm, either to release overwhelming feelings or to become numb.

Over time, their alarm system is hijacked as they become increasingly tolerant of high levels of fear and threat to the point that everything and everyone feels threatening, making it hard to recognise real danger. In addition, they can become irritable, angry, hostile, and aggressive. As they adapt to a constant state of hyper-arousal they are less able to discriminate between safety and danger, and see danger in things which non-survivors would find safe and relaxing.

As these overwhelming emotions and intense bodily sensations are experienced as confusing and do not make sense, they are hard to tolerate or manage. This can lead to desperate attempts at finding external sources of self-soothing such as substance misuse or self-harm. As hyper-arousal is exhausting and cannot be sustained long term, many survivors resort to numbing to blunt overwhelming emotions which can lead to dissociation, detachment, and a restricted range of emotions.

While hypo-arousal is a way of tolerating intolerable emotions it does not allow survivors to select which emotions get turned down, which means that all feelings and sensations, even pleasurable ones, are erased or suppressed.

In addition, hypo-arousal prevents survivors from being aware of actual danger or threat in their environment, making them more vulnerable to further abuse or harm. It is important to note that while hyper- and hypo-arousal can lead to increased vulnerability to danger and lack of emotional regulation, there are some adaptive elements to these instinctual reactions.

The increased level of alertness associated with hyper-arousal can lead to quick-wittedness and an ability to engage in mental acrobatics such as mental arithmetic or verbal ability. Similarly, hypo-arousal in shutting down emotions allows some survivors to live in their head and develop cognitive and intellectual capacities resulting in high academic attainment and increased career opportunities. Such escape into intellectual retreat acts as a distraction and relief from the abuse which allows the survivor to feel less helpless and powerless, and take pride in their abilities. Survivors who are able to channel hyper-arousal or hypo-arousal in this way are often highly successful in their careers but at a huge emotional cost, especially in their personal relationships.

Emotional dysregulation is likely to be triggered by trauma reminders, or when there is no source of comfort or when in proximity to the person who caused the harm. As the child is unable to access an external source of comfort they cannot develop the inner resources to regulate their emotions. This leads them to seek external sources of comfort to numb emotions such as alcohol, drugs, food, work, sex, or relationships.

Alternatively, they may engage in thrill seeking or risky behaviours such as extreme sports, unsafe sexual encounters, or stimulants to re-experience high states of arousal and the rush of adrenaline in order to 'feel alive'. As many of these compensatory regulatory strategies are accompanied by shame and humiliation, it can trigger the anger and rage suppressed during the abuse and result in hostile, aggressive, or violent behaviour. While this is a way of discharging deeply buried emotions it can alienate others, or potentially lead to antisocial behaviour or criminal offences. Ultimately it is these reactions to trauma that impact on a range of mental and physical health difficulties, as well as relationship problems.

In addition, trauma reactions prevent many survivors from reaching their full potential as all their energy is consumed in getting through each day. It also makes it extremely hard to live in a terrifying present in which they are forced to relive the trauma or remain on constant hyper-alert and be prepared for danger in the future. Unless they are able to learn skills to regulate their emotions and expand their window of tolerance (Siegel, 1999), survivors become trapped in an endless cycle of hyper- or hypo-arousal. In addition, prolonged sleep disturbances such as nightmares, night-time flashbacks, night terrors, night-time panic attacks, and parasomnias can lead to a range of daytime symptoms such as exhaustion, poor concentration, and disorientation, and in some cases exacerbate dissociative symptoms, especially depersonalisation and derealisation.

Expanding the survivor's window of tolerance allows them to develop a degree of control and emotional self-regulation, and the skills to calm themselves when arousal rises to upper limits and goes into hyper-arousal, or to feel when arousal drops to low levels leading to hypo-arousal or dissociation. While the capacity for emotional self-regulation is usually learnt in early attachment relationships, it is hijacked or narrowed when exposed to repeated trauma and SSA. The impact of the lack of emotional self-regulation is not just a difficulty in regulating emotions, but also affects the ability to relate to others, as well as the capacity for attention, concentration, and focus, all of which can negatively influence belief systems and increase emotional distress.

Dissociation

As we touched on in the previous chapter in relation to children, dissociation allows the survivor to numb their body and mind, and this also applies to adults. In this, they erase somatic sensations and bodily experiences, as well as emotions and feelings, including positive ones such as pleasure or joy. As they become more alienated from emotions and sensations they begin to live in the safety of their head rather than their body. In deleting their body and accompanying somatic sensation they have difficulty in their awareness and expression of somatic feelings and sensations which can lead to a lack of somatic literacy and alexisomia. As they increasingly avoid emotions these cannot be processed and will persist and demand attention, trapping the survivor into a relentless cycle of hyper- and hypo-arousal and confusion. This in turn prevents them from identifying and expressing feelings as they are unable to find words to represent these, leading to lack of emotional literacy, or alexithymia. This can be falsely perceived as cold and unfeeling, rather than the reality which is that overwhelming feelings of terror have rendered them speechless and voiceless.

Persistent and chronic dissociation can lead to depersonalisation in which a survivor's sense of self and identity becomes confused, and in which they are unsure about who they are or experience their body as unreal, changing, or dissolving. Depersonalisation is often the most common form of dissociation seen in clinical practice, albeit poorly recognised or understood by both client and practitioner (Sanderson, 2004, 2022). Many survivors become so estranged from themselves that they do not recognise themselves when looking in the mirror or looking at photographs or images of themselves. As a result they feel lost and confused about their identity and who they are. They can also become detached from their body and have out-of-body experiences, or feel as though they are watching themselves in a dream or film rather than actually experiencing what is happening to them (see Table 7.1 for more on dissociative symptoms).

Table 7.1 Range of dissociative symptoms

Dissociative symptom	Presentation	Lived experience quotes
Amnesia	No memories of the past or the trauma Amnesia in day-to-day life, memory lapses of seconds, minutes, or hours Loss of skills such as language, reading, or writing	'it didn't happen to me', 'it didn't hurt', 'I don't remember', 'I don't care that it happened', 'it doesn't really matter', 'I am fine, there is nothing wrong with me', 'I didn't do anything', 'I don't know'
Depersonalisation	Estrangement from self, feeling strange, unreal, or robotic. Often feel detached, or as though they are an outside observer of their own thoughts, feelings, sensations, body, or actions, out-of-body experiences Deleting the body	'my body has disappeared', 'my body is not mine', 'something takes over my body and I have no control over it', 'I am lost', 'I can't see', 'I can't hear', 'I can't control my body', 'I am dead inside'
Derealisation	Estrangement from surroundings in which others, objects, or the world are experienced as unreal – dreamlike, distant, foggy, lifeless, colourless, or visually and time distorted Feeling detached or removed from surroundings	'it's all a dream', 'it's not real', 'other people are not real, or like robots', 'I feel like I am floating away', 'I feel like I am drowning', 'it's all foggy and hazy'

Dissociative symptom	Presentation	Lived experience quotes
Identity confusion	Inner struggle of self and identity; identity alteration – acting like a different person, false self, compliant or good child Feeling as though there are different people inside, losing control to 'someone else' inside them, acting like different people, speaking in different voices with different ages	'we don't like this', 'they are telling me I have to do this', 'I don't know who I am', 'it wasn't me, it was them telling me what to do', 'I didn't do it, they did'
Dissociative identity disorder	Disruption of a person's identity, where a person has two or more distinct identities	'the voices are there all the time', 'the voices tell me to say and do things', 'the voice tells me not to trust anyone'

Severe dissociation can also lead to derealisation in which the world seems unreal, where the familiar is unfamiliar, where they or their friends become unreal or turn into robots and objects appear to change in shape, size, or colour. The overall experience is saturated with vague and dreamlike states which are typically described by survivors as like being in a haze or fog.

Some survivors may become so dissociated that they experience structural dissociation, in which the sense of self splits into two distinct states: one is what Van der Hart et al. (2004) name as the Apparently Normal Personality, which is highly functional. The other is the Emotional Personality, or Traumatised Personality, in which there are multiple splits (see also Boon et al., 2011; Steele et al., 2017; Fisher, 2021).

When a survivor becomes so dissociated, they can develop dissociative identity disorder, where the mind 'splits off' parts that it is unable to cope with and which go on to form into several parts (see Chapter 6).

The symptoms of dissociation are often behind mood swings or personality shifts, forgetfulness, dreamlike states, inattention, or memory loss for periods of time. It can be frightening and distressing for a survivor if they can't remember where they were or what they were doing for periods of time – hours, days, or sometimes weeks. In addition, dissociation often underpins other mental health problems such as depression, bi-polar disorder, anxiety disorders, personality disorders, self-harm, OCD, sleep deprivation, and addictions.

Memory

Trauma and lack of emotional regulation also impacts on the processing of memories which can lead to memory difficulties. Survivors commonly experience flashbacks, nightmares, intrusive memories, and images which are often disconnected from the abuse experience or do not make sense. As these intrusive images and flashbacks are so overwhelming they are blocked from conscious awareness and cannot be processed, continuing to remain alive or 'online' (Sanderson, 2022). This results in a stream of distressing memories that remain raw and unprocessed and cannot be stored or integrated into long-term memory. In addition, memories that aren't processed cannot be accessed verbally or through conscious or deliberate recall and differ significantly from normal 'verbally accessible memory' (VAM) which is organised, time tagged, and can be integrated and updated with new information.

In contrast, traumatic memories are fragmented and frozen in time, and often emerge involuntarily in response to trauma cues. These memories are often non-verbal and represent 'situationally accessible memory' (SAM), in that they are triggered automatically outside of conscious awareness through flashbacks or nightmares (Sanderson, 2022). They often consist of feelings, sensations, and behavioural responses that were present at the time of the trauma and contain intense fear responses and emotions which were sealed off. As they are not accessible to conscious awareness they cannot be processed and remain etched on the brain and in the body to return in the presence of internal or external cues associated with the trauma. For some survivors they can persist as recurring thoughts and ruminations, or constant replaying of the trauma which cannot be turned off.

The lack of VAMs, and the predominance of SAMs, means that survivors live in a constant state of threat with little or no understanding as to why they feel terrified. In addition, uncontrollable flashbacks and intrusive memories which have no context can make survivors feel as though they are going crazy. It is important for survivors to know that these are typical traumatic memory reactions and that they can be worked through once they have mastered emotional self-regulation and are in a safe environment to explore the traumatic memories and create a coherent narrative of the abuse experience.

Triggers

The over-activated threat detection system means that survivors' neuroception of risk and safety is intensified in order to assess whether people and situations are safe, dangerous, or life threatening. While this occurs outside of conscious awareness it means that survivors are more sensitised to external and internal threats, and become easily triggered in the presence of danger and trauma-related cues. To help survivors to feel more in control of intrusive sensations and memories, they need to be able to identify the external and internal triggers that activate hyper- or hypo-arousal, flashbacks, intrusive memories, or dissociative states. In addition, it is important for survivors to be aware of triggers so that they can plan ways of managing these. This is especially the case when the survivor has no conscious memory of the SSA but is suddenly flooded by bodily sensations or flashbacks.

Mental Health

Trauma reactions give rise to a range of symptoms that impact on mental and physical health as well as relationship problems. As many of these reactions occur outside of conscious awareness, survivors are often unaware of how they link to their abuse experience. This, alongside their confusion and fear that they are going mad, makes it hard for them to give a context to their symptoms, which can lead to misinterpretation and misdiagnosis. In order to ensure that survivors are understood and able to gain access to the right support and therapeutic help, it is critical to have an understanding of the long-term effects and the range of symptoms associated with SSA to have a better understanding of survivors and respond to them more empathically and compassionately.

Common signs are being on edge, irritable, unpredictable, impulsive, zoned out, unresponsive, lethargic, or emotionless, and mood swings. Some survivors become highly suspicious, hostile, defensive, angry, aggressive, or controlling. In contrast, others become overly compliant, submissive, passive, or overly trusting, and constantly engage in testing behaviours such as rebuffing or being critical. The pervasive chronic shame, self-loathing, and self-hatred can lead to withdrawal and isolation, or compulsive behaviours such as obsessive thoughts and rumination, perfectionism, and over-achieving. A history of CSA and SSA is highly correlated with prolonged alcohol and drug misuse, self-harm, suicidal ideation, and suicidal behaviours, as well as a range of physical mental health issues. Sibling sexual abuse also impacts on relationship difficulties, including fear of closeness and intimacy, sexual difficulties, sexual confusion, and compulsive sexual behaviour. The betrayal of trust in SSA leads to deep-seated fears of being hurt, rejection, abandonment, and being let down again. This can lead to becoming either highly avoidant or highly dependent on others, with lack of autonomy and self-efficacy.

Many survivors find it hard to trust, or trust too quickly in the hope that this time it will be different, and will often test others to see whether they can be trusted. This is often done through hostility, anger, and pushing away of others which is driven by fear rather than aggression, and must be understood as such. Many survivors want to be loved and cared for but are afraid of this, as love and care means being abused and hurt. In addition, as many survivors cannot accept let alone like themselves, they find it hard to believe that others might like or care for them. Practitioners need to be mindful of this and respond in an empathic and compassionate way rather than reject the survivor.

This can also be the case in survivors who appear to be high functioning, fiercely independent, or grandiose and arrogant. Such survivors often reject or devalue any help that is offered by shifting their sense of shame away from themselves onto others. It is critical to persevere in the presence of such behaviours to show the survivor that they will not reject him or her. Understanding these signs will be invaluable to understand the symptoms typically associated with survivors of SSA.

Depression

There are many causes of depression and it is very common for survivors to suffer crippling bouts of depression during their lives, especially if memories of SSA are triggered. Common triggers for female survivors are pregnancy, the need for intimate examinations, giving birth, the gender of the child, or the child reaching the age when the survivor experienced SSA. Male survivors also report an increase in intrusive memories and depression when they become fathers.

Male and female survivors who wanted to have children often develop depression later in life as a result of not having had children. An unrecognised history of SSA can make the treatment of depression more difficult and hinder recovery unless there is some trauma-focused therapy.

Anxiety

Anxiety disorders arise due to heightened levels of anxiety which appear generalised, or 'free floating', unless a link to SSA is made. Anxiety and panic attacks are common, and typically resemble the fear and panic experienced during the SSA as the body re-experiences trauma symptoms. Most anxiety disorders can be understood in the context of trauma symptoms and it helps if a survivor can identify potential links rather than believe they are irrational.

Avoiding intrusive memories or thoughts can lead to agoraphobia or claustrophobia, while avoiding places, people, or objects associated with the SSA can explain a range of other phobic reactions, and it is important to explore these sensitively. Anxiety and panic attacks can make it difficult to be visible or seen, to concentrate and study, or to work – all of which can further erode self-confidence and restrict activities.

Not wanting to be visible, shame, and fear of others can lead to chronic social anxiety in which the survivor is unable to engage with others, and fears leaving the safety of their home or only going out late at night or early in the morning when they are less likely to be seen by others.

Some survivors may have difficulty sleeping, or need to sleep with the light on, and may wake up panicky or depressed. These anxiety-based disorders affect not only a survivor but partners and other family members who may find themselves restricted by the survivor's anxieties and fears. To manage these some survivors resort to self-medication to regulate their mood or emotional states through the use of substances such as alcohol, drugs, medication, or food, or through excessive exercise, work, shopping, sex, or relationships.

Obsessive Compulsive Behaviours

In order to feel more in control, some survivors may develop obsessive compulsive behaviours to keep terrifying fears and thoughts at bay, while others brood and believe themselves to be at risk of harming others. Many OCD symptoms can be linked to SSA such as fear of contamination and hand washing, tidiness and neatness to reduce internal chaos, or checking behaviours to quell fears of harm or intrusion, or counting to distract from overwhelming terror, or rhythmic touching or striking to self-soothe.

A survivor may engage in endless brooding, or mental compulsions, in which negative and shameful thoughts about harming others or having committed appalling crimes are repeatedly replayed in their head (Sanderson, 2022). The rituals seen in OCD and mental compulsions can be exhausting and time consuming, making it hard for a survivor to engage in other activities, go to work, or live life fully. The treatment of OCD is often complicated but can be made easier if there is a link identified between the symptoms, a history of SSA, and shame.

Eating Disorders

Eating disorders are often seen in survivors, who use food to either numb feelings or self-comfort, such as in compulsive eating, or binge eating to put on weight so as to become unattractive and avoid sexual attention. Anorexia is often a way of gaining a semblance of control over a deep sense of powerlessness, or to avoid the onset of puberty as it heralds emergent sexuality and sexual feelings, romantic or sexual relationships and the possibility of pregnancy, or simply a wish to die. While eating disorders can occur for a variety of reasons, they are highly correlated with CSA and SSA. This is also seen in bulimia and orthorexia nervosa which is characterised by an extreme obsession with eating 'pure' food. While not all eating disorders have their origins in SSA, it is important to explore this as a possibility to ensure that this is addressed during treatment.

Self-Harm

This is strongly linked to SSA and can range from self-neglect and lack of self-care through to cutting, gouging, and burning. Self-harm is primarily a coping mechanism to either release emotional and psychological pain, or as a way to numb overwhelming feelings through the release of endorphins in the brain that anaesthetise that pain and give rise to a feeling of euphoria. A survivor may engage in self-harm, either as a form of self-hatred and self-punishment or as a compulsive re-enactment of the experience of CSA.

It is crucial to explore and develop an understanding of the link between self-harm and self-injury and its relationship to SSA rather than dismiss it as a form of attention seeking so that they can find alternative ways of regulating their emotions. Practitioners must also be aware that self-harm is primarily a survival strategy and as such quite distinct from attempted suicide. Some survivors, particularly males, engage in self-harm through compulsive risk taking – extreme sports, unsafe sex, thrill-seeking, heavy drug or alcohol misuse, or gambling – or excessive exercise or work.

Self-harm through the use of alcohol, drugs, food, gambling, or sex all have the capacity to induce dissociative states to numb pain or overwhelming feelings. Initially these may be used as a form of self-medication, which with regular use can lead to dependency or addiction. As addictions and self-harm are also a source of shame, many survivors feel even more overwhelmed thereby increasing the need to self-medicate and getting lost in a never-ending cycle of addiction. In this the original need to self-medicate becomes lost as the primary focus is on the addiction. This is often reinforced by health professionals who concentrate on treating the addiction rather than linking the addiction to a history of trauma and working through this.

Suicidal Ideation and Behaviour

Many survivors of SSA report a history of suicidal thoughts and repeated suicide attempts. What is not known is how many survivors succeed without having revealed the secret of their abuse. As many survivors already feel that they are living a 'psychological death' the thought or act of suicide is a source of comfort, as it would release them from their distress. The risk of suicide is also elevated in 'dual status' siblings, and siblings who committed SSA.

A survivor may not actually want to take their life but wish to have some temporary relief from their pain, or go to sleep and never wake up. As a result they may over-medicate in order to dull or deaden the pain they experience and risk over-dosing. Young male survivors are most at risk of suicide often by engaging in life-threatening forms of risk-taking behaviour.

Somatisation and Physical Illnesses

Survivors of SSA may experience physical harm such as genital and anal damage, sexually transmitted diseases, pelvic inflammatory disease, gynaecological problems, and reduced fertility. They may develop chronic pain either as a result of their injuries or through somatisation and the physical expression of emotional pain. This can result in a range of unexplained illnesses such as recurrent chest pains, breathing problems, irritable bowel symptoms, and autoimmune disorders, as well as chronic fatigue syndrome and loss of vitality.

Sleep Disturbances

Traumatised clients tend to experience more severe sleep disturbances such as night-time flashbacks, trauma-related nightmares, night terrors, and night-time panic attacks. While many survivors are able to armour themselves during the day to keep distressing thoughts, feelings, and memories at bay through distractions, when their armour is removed at night what was kept at bay is unleashed, leading to a sense of dread at going to sleep, insomnia, disrupted sleep, disturbing dreams and nightmares, and night-time panic attacks. In addition, clients whose sleep is consistently compromised will suffer from sleep exhaustion, impaired cognitive and executive functioning, daytime dissociative states, in particular depersonalisation, as well as a compromised immune system and concomitant physical health problems, all of which exacerbate trauma symptoms.

Alcohol and Drugs

Current research on the impact of early childhood adverse experiences on later mental and physical health, and increased vulnerability to addiction, includes a number of studies which found that ACEs such as physical, emotional, and sexual abuse, neglect, and growing up with domestic abuse increase the risk of addiction (Felitti et al., 1998). Individuals who have experienced more than four ACEs are seven times more likely to become addicted to alcohol, ten times more likely to be at risk of intravenous drug addiction, and 12 times more likely to have attempted suicide. This research has led to a deeper understanding of addiction as a form of self-medication to manage painful experiences (Khantzian & Albanese, 2008) and attempts at emotional regulation (Maté, 2009; Van der Kolk, 2015; One in Four, 2019; Sanderson, 2019).

Alcohol, drugs, food, and sex, as well as self-harm, all have the capacity to induce dissociative states to numb pain or overwhelming feelings. Initially these may be used as a form of self-medication, which with regular use can lead to dependency or addiction. As addictions and self-harm are also a source of shame, many survivors feel even more overwhelmed thereby increasing the need to self-medicate and getting lost in a never-ending cycle of addiction. In this the original need to self-medicate becomes lost as the primary focus is on the addiction. This is often reinforced by health professionals who concentrate on treating the addiction rather than linking the addiction to a history of trauma and working through that instead.

Psychosocial Impact

A history of SSA can make survivors more vulnerable to revictimisation as they are unable to say no or set boundaries in relationships and risk further sexual or domestic abuse. In addition they may have an increased tolerance threshold for being abused as they will have normalised this. In not being able to assert themselves or express their needs in case they are abandoned they become submissive and compliant.

Survivors who protect themselves by being hostile and aggressive are at increased risk of antisocial behaviour, especially if they are dependent on the use of drugs or alcohol. This can lead to being lured into criminal activities and the risk of custodial sentences.

Culture, Marginalisation, and Intersectionality

When SSA occurs within an environment of racism, poverty, class, cultural discrimination, or marginalisation on the basis of gender and gender identity, it is crucial to acknowledge how these intersect with the SSA. Practitioners need to be aware of how such intersectionality impacts on the survivor and adopt a culturally aware approach alongside cultural sensitivity and cultural humility.

This will allow them to have a deeper understanding of the impact of SSA and to focus attention on what happened to the survivor rather than focusing on what is wrong with them or pathologising them. It is also important to acknowledge the range of strengths and positive resources which survivors acquire in order to survive their abuse and to validate these in order to counterbalance the deficits. It is important to identify resources and coping skills and to build on these rather than focus solely on the negative impact of SSA as these will lead to the empowerment of the survivor throughout their healing process.

The following chapter will look at how these long-term effects impact on the survivor's sense of self and self-perception, and how they can lead to enduring personality changes in order to adapt to threat responses. It will also explore how the fear of being in a relationship can lead to tumultuous and labile relationships, including therapeutic ones.

Further Reading

Boon, S., Steele, K., & van der Hart, O. (2011). *Coping with trauma-related dissociation: Skills training for patients and therapists*. W.W. Norton.

Dell, P.F., & O'Neill, J.A. (2015). *Dissociation and the dissociative disorders: DSM-5 and beyond*. Routledge.

Caffaro, J.V., & Conn-Caffaro, A. (1998). *Sibling abuse trauma: Assessment and intervention strategies for children, families and adults*. Routledge.

Fisher, J. (2017). *Healing the fragmented selves of trauma survivors*. Routledge.

Kezelman, C.A., & Stavropoulos, P.A. (2020). *Practice guidelines for identifying and treating complex trauma related dissociation*. Blue Knot Foundation.

McCartan, K., Anning, A., & Qureshi, E. (2021). *The impact of sibling sexual abuse on adults who were harmed as children*. UWE, Bristol Research Report.

Sanderson, C. (2013). *Counselling skills for working with trauma*. Jessica Kingsley Publishers.

Sanderson, C. (2015). *Responding to survivors of child sexual abuse: A pocket guide for professionals, partners, families and friends*. One in Four.

Sanderson, C. (2017). *Dissociation and dissociative disorders: Advice for adults suffering with dissociation and those working with them*. One in Four.

Sanderson, C. (2019). *Numbing the pain: A pocket guide for professionals supporting survivors of childhood sexual abuse and addiction*. One in Four.

Sanderson, C. (2022). *The warrior within: A One in Four handbook to aid recovery for survivors of childhood sexual abuse and violence* (4th edn). One in Four.

Steele, K., Boon, S., & van der Hart (2017). Treating trauma-related dissociation: A practical integrated approach. W.W. Norton.

van der Hart, O., Nijenhuis, E., & Steele, K. (2006). *The haunted self: Structural dissociation and the treatment of chronic traumatisation*. W.W. Norton.

Van der Kolk, B. (2015). *The body keeps the score: Mind, brain and body in the transformation of trauma*. Penguin Books.

CHAPTER 8

The Intrapersonal and Relational Effects of Sibling Sexual Abuse in Adult Survivors

This chapter will look at how the long-term effects of SSA impact on the adult survivor's sense of self, self-perception, and shame, and how this can lead to enduring personality changes in order to adapt to threat responses and how these are often mislabelled or misdiagnosed as personality disorders, in particular borderline personality disorder (emotionally unstable personality disorder). It will also explore how the fear of being in a relationship can lead to tumultuous and labile relationships, including the therapeutic one, as the survivor struggles between yearning to be close and fearing closeness. This leads to the need to regulate closeness through approach and avoid behaviours, or re-enactments of interactions with their sibling.

Sense of Self and Self-Identity
Many survivors of SSA experience a profound loss of self and self-identity, which leaves them feeling lost or broken, as though there is something missing. They commonly feel different to everyone else and report feeling dirty, defective, worthless, and unlovable, which negatively impacts on their self-esteem and self-confidence.

The lack of self necessitates wearing a mask to cover up the inner emptiness and to pretend to be normal. Conversely, some survivors try to stay under the radar by becoming chameleon-like and blending in, or they make themselves invisible so as not to draw attention to themselves. While this allows them to adapt to whatever others expect of them, it undermines the development of a cohesive sense of self.

As the self becomes more and more fragmented the survivor loses a sense of stability of the self which leads to self-doubt and the inability to trust themselves. Many survivors fear making any decisions in case they get it wrong and as a result lose any sense of self-agency.

In the absence of a core self-identity some survivors become vulnerable to adopting a victim or survivor identity which can be self-limiting. This can hold them hostage to defining themselves solely as survivors of SSA, rather than seeing it as something that happened to them which does not define who they are or the whole of their self.

Some survivors also become confused about their gender identity and sexuality (see the case of Beryl later in this chapter). Male survivors of sexual violence often feel that their masculinity has been compromised, culminating in a loss of confidence in their 'maleness'. This commonly results in a recurring need to 'prove' their masculinity through hyper-masculine behaviour, or toxic masculinity. Simon who was made to dress up in girls' clothing and told to behave in a 'feminine' way while being raped by his older brother became utterly confused about his gender identity and what it meant to be male or female. He associated masculinity with the abuse of power and sexual assault and femininity with being passive and submissive (see Simon's case later in this chapter). This gender and identity confusion persisted throughout his adolescence, making it hard to have any sense of his sexual orientation or pursue any romantic or sexual relationships. The concomitant sense of shame can lead many survivors to withdraw from others and compound their isolation and lack of belongingness.

Shame

Survivors of SSA often become prisoners of shame. This is not just due to the shaming experiences during the abuse such as feeling sexually aroused or not having defended themselves more, but also includes being made to feel ashamed for basic human needs, or feeling defective. Such shame is often elicited when they have sexual feelings as adults, or when engaging in sexual intimacy. This is confusing as they want to be sexually intimate with their partner, but they also fear feeling ashamed. To manage such confusion many survivors dissociate during sexual intimacy and go on autopilot during the sexual encounter. Once they have orgasmed or the sexual activity ceases they come out of dissociation and are flooded with shame, disgust, and self-loathing.

Such self-loathing and negative evaluations and feelings about the self lead to corrosive self-critical thoughts. Many survivors become shame-prone and highly sensitised to shame, and persistently seek confirmation of their 'shameworthiness' (One in Four, 2015; Sanderson, 2022) often by perpetuating shame through shame-based ruminations, or seeking out or engaging in shame-based behaviours.

Shame proneness is predicated on the awareness of 'self as bad' and 'self as inadequate', which leads to becoming highly sensitised to shaming experiences, real or imagined. This is typically seen in acute sensitivity to shaming aspects through the use of language or non-verbal communication such as body language which suggest that the self is worthless.

Survivors may also experience secondary shame wherein they feel shame for their feelings, such as sadness or anxiety, their emotional reactions such as dependency needs or vulnerability, or feeling ashamed. To defend against shame survivors may withdraw by hiding or isolating themselves, physically or psychologically. Alternatively they may attack the self through negative talk and beliefs about the self, or self-shaming behaviours. Some survivors use self-deprecating humour to manage their shame in an attempt to stay connected to others.

Some survivors avoid the feeling of shame by numbing it through the use of drugs or alcohol, or by covering it up with perfectionism, excessive pride, arrogance, grandiosity, or narcissism. It is helpful to recognise that narcissistic traits such as arrogance and grandiosity are compensatory strategies to mask shame and an effective way of keeping people at bay, which reduces the risk of the shame being exposed. A further defence against shame is to attack others, wherein the focus of shame is deflected away from the survivor and projected onto others. This is seen in undermining others, bullying, abuse, and sexual violence.

Negative Self-Perception, Self-Thoughts, and Self-Talk

The shame and debased self-identity have a significant impact on the survivor's perception of self. This is seen in feelings of self-loathing and feeling like 'damaged goods', and a sense of being so unlovable that others will be repulsed by them. This negative view of the self is often supported by negative beliefs about the self and concomitant negative self-talk. These negative self-perceptions can lead to negative automatic thoughts, self-criticism, and ruminations, which can be so corrosive that some survivors feel that they have no right to exist. This can increase dependency on others to value them and shore up their self-esteem, which further reinforces a sense of shame and powerlessness.

Negative thoughts and beliefs are often inflamed by trauma and heightened anxiety, and are more likely to consist of biased thinking as the person is in survival mode and not able to fully engage in objective cognitive processing. As a result survivors are more vulnerable to misjudgements that tend to reinforce fears or anxieties and prolong pain and perpetuate negative beliefs and distorted thinking. Sometimes these are so habitual that they become automatic and seem to occur outside conscious awareness. This is often due to internalised distorted perceptions inserted by the harming sibling which have been incorporated into the survivor's belief system.

Negative self-beliefs such as 'I am to blame', 'I am bad', 'I am worthless', 'I am unlovable', 'I am a failure', or 'I am dirty and filthy' infect the self-identity and can lead to filtering the world through the harming sibling's eyes, voice, and actions, and become so deeply embedded that the survivor may not even be aware of their negative thoughts or their impact.

This censorious internal critic serves to constantly undermine the survivor and sabotages any capacity for self-esteem.

Some survivors engage in endless rumination, or covert compulsions in which negative and shameful thoughts about harming others or having committed appalling crimes are repeatedly replayed in their head. These self-deprecating ruminations are extremely exhausting and time consuming, making it hard for the survivor to engage in other activities, go to work, or live life fully.

To compensate for perceived flaws many survivors impose unrealistic expectations on themselves, leading to a need to be perfect to compensate for their perceived deficiencies. As the expectations in perfectionist thinking and behaviour are unrealistic and virtually impossible to achieve, the survivor is inevitably destined to fail. This reinforces the sense of failure, guilt, and self-criticism, and the cycle continues.

Enduring Personality Changes

Survivors who have experienced sexual abuse are vulnerable to being diagnosed with a personality disorder, in particular borderline personality disorder, also known as emotionally unstable personality disorder.

Such diagnoses have become not only stigmatising but also a 'dustbin diagnosis' for people who are perceived as 'attention seeking', non-compliant, or who behave 'badly', persistently self-harm, or abuse substances.

It is essential that practitioners recognise that a prolonged history of SSA leads to enduring personality changes, and that many of the symptoms are a result of trauma reactions and PTSD rather than attention-seeking. While it is true that survivors with borderline personality disorder can be challenging to work with as they are often suspicious or mistrustful, and who switch between being needy and dependent to being avoidant or hostile, it is important that these symptoms are seen as accommodations to living under threat and trauma rather than a personality disorder. Such survivors require a safe, empathic, and consistent relationship with compassionate and firm boundaries in which they begin to trust.

Living under threat for prolonged periods of time can result in enduring personality changes (Herman, 1992, 2023) characteristic of 'enduring personality change after catastrophic experience' (International Statistical Classification of Diseases and Related Health Problems, 11th Revision (ICD-11); World Health Organization, 2018) which are characterised by a hostile or distrustful attitude toward the world, social withdrawal, feelings of emptiness or hopelessness, a chronic feeling of 'being on edge' as if constantly threatened, and estrangement from self and environment, somatisation, self-injurious behaviours, sexual difficulties, and enduring guilt and shame. These symptoms are in essence adaptations to living under threat in which there is no escape which necessitates changes to the personality in order to survive pervasive threat (Johnstone & Boyle, 2018; Boyle & Johnstone, 2020).

When these symptoms coexist with other trauma symptoms such as hyper-arousal, mood swings, inflexible patterns of thought and behaviour, and relationship difficulties, these personality traits are commonly mislabelled and misdiagnosed as personality disorders, in particular borderline personality disorder and antisocial personality disorder. Similarly, survivors who are highly dissociative and experience visual or auditory perceptual disturbances or hallucinations may be misdiagnosed with psychotic disorders.

Many survivors diagnosed with personality disorders may never have experienced a genuinely caring relationship, and in providing this professionals can create an opportunity to develop a relationship which allows them to heal. To do this, practitioners need to respond to the survivor's obvious distress rather than provocative behaviour, be patient and not personalise attacks, instead seeing these as 'anger born of fear' rather than deliberate aggression.

Relationships and Lack of Relational Worth

Many survivors are scared to be themselves for fear of being seen as unlovable, worthless, flawed, or powerless. These survivors describe themselves as being trapped in two emotional worlds, one of anger and despair, and the other of terror and shame, which they have to conceal. They are afraid to be themselves, or show their true feelings or needs for fear of being seen as bad or selfish, or fear of further rejection or abandonment. This can lead to compliant and people-pleasing behaviour as they hide their feelings, thoughts, or needs by adopting a false self, and living a double life in order to stay safe and protect the true self (Sanderson, 2015, 2016).

The betrayal of trust and inappropriate boundaries in SSA mean that many survivors experience relationship difficulties. Many find it hard to trust others as they fear further betrayal or abandonment; some become overly trusting, while others avoid relationships at all costs. This is due to them feeling that relationships are a source of fear and terror rather than places of safety or solace. While the survivor wants to be loved and cared for they don't know how to permit that, as for them love is equated with harm and abuse.

As a result they get caught in a never-ending cycle of attempts to be close to others followed by pushing them away, which is both confusing and exhausting for the survivor and their partner. In addition, self-hatred and lack of self-acceptance means that a survivor may become suspicious of anyone who claims to love or care for them. To protect themselves they may be compelled to keep people at bay, often through anger or hostility. This anger is typically due to fear rather than aggression, and requires empathy and compassion rather than judgement or punishment.

A survivor may fear closeness and intimacy so much that they are unable to form any significant relationships and remain alone and isolated throughout their lives, which becomes a source of shame and proof of their unlovability and worthlessness. Sexual abuse in childhood forces survivors to be submissive and compliant which typically translates into people-pleasing in adulthood. As a result they may tolerate behaviours that are adversive as they are not sure how to set boundaries – either because they expect no better or they believe they deserve to be treated badly. Not being able to say no to disrespectful or aggressive behaviour makes them more vulnerable to re-victimisation or being enticed into abusive relationships.

Many survivors believe that the only way to avoid being hurt or abandoned is to please others, or rescue and fix them. This renders them more vulnerable to abusive relationships which are characterised by submission or domination, or violence and coercive control. This translates into elements of so-called 'co-dependency' in which the individual 'needs to be needed' and is often enmeshed with 'people who need to dominate'. The unpredictability of relationships and fear of being betrayed leads to detachment from others. As the connection to others weakens, it reinforces the sense of isolation and aloneness, while increasing the need to connect to others, and the shame in not being able to do so.

Survivors who fear dependency and who are excessively fiercely independent tend to mask their needs and vulnerability, and try to control the behaviour of others or re-enact controlling and abusive patterns from childhood. In order to manage such highly stressful and chaotic relationships, survivors need to learn to express their needs without shame and be able to set healthy boundaries and say no without fear.

The fear of closeness can also be seen in other relationships such as family members, siblings, work colleagues, and professional relationships. It is crucial to link this to the SSA and promote safety and trust in which survivors can learn to trust others, rather than avoid them.

Some survivors may also experience relationship difficulties with their children by becoming over-protective, especially when their child reaches the age when they themselves were first abused, which can impact their parenting. While many survivors seek therapeutic support when they become parents in order to ensure that their experience of sexual abuse does not influence their parenting, most survivors fear not being able to protect their child or children from being sexually abused. Many survivors are triggered when they become parents which can lead to reactivation of the trauma and returning trauma symptoms. Some survivors may find it hard to display affection to their children or neglect them by avoiding appropriate physical contact or routine hygiene care. This is not due to lack of love or care but is driven by a deep-seated fear of being perceived as abusing them, or compelled to touch them in a sexual way. This does not necessarily mean that their children are at risk of sexual harm, rather it is a reflection of overwhelming fear of physical contact and touch, and what that might lead to as it did in the original SSA.

Alternatively some survivors become over-protective of their children by over-identifying with them and becoming enmeshed with the child. As a result they may make the child anxious about engaging with others or forming friendships in case they are sexually abused. In instilling a fear of others the survivor inadvertently impedes the development of healthy relationship skills. Thus the child may become socially anxious and isolated as they sense there is something wrong without knowing why. This can lead to a fear of future relationships and a pervasive anxiety that being close to someone will harm them.

Intimacy and Sexual Challenges

Many survivors experience a range of sexual challenges ranging from suppressed sexuality and lack of sexual interest through to compulsive sexual behaviour and compulsive masturbation. These difficulties must not be judged as they often represent aspects of the abuse in which avoiding sex is a way of saying no which they were not able to in childhood, while compulsive sexual behaviour may be due to heightened sexual sensitisation due to developmentally premature sexual excitation. As the survivor feels compelled to re-enact or relive aspects of the sexual abuse through masturbation or certain sexual actions, the sexual activity is rarely experienced as pleasurable or satisfying as it is suffused with self-loathing, shame, and disgust. Survivors who dissociate during sexual intimacy may suddenly come back into the present after orgasming and will be suffused with anger and rage and attack their partner, which can be inordinately confusing for both. Other survivors will cry uncontrollably and inconsolably throughout the sexual interaction. It is helpful that partners have access to psychoeducation and support so that they are able to understand the survivor and remain connected to them (Sanderson, 2013, 2022).

Many of the sexual challenges faced by survivors are due to a crippling sense of shame and confusion about sexuality, especially if they were sexually aroused during the abuse. Survivors often misinterpret sexual arousal during SSA as evidence that they must have enjoyed it or wanted the abuse to happen. This leads to self-blame, making it harder to legitimise it as abuse. It is important that survivors and professionals recognise that sexual responses during abuse are a normal physiological response of the body unrelated to sexual enjoyment or desire which can be intensified by high levels of adrenaline caused by fear and anxiety.

A survivor may also experience confusion about their sexual orientation, with some avoiding sex altogether. A survivor attracted to people of the same sex may worry that the abuse 'made them' gay, lesbian, or bisexual, and consequently can feel bad about their sexual feelings, while heterosexual male survivors abused by men may worry that their abuser thought they were gay and chose to abuse them as a result. This may lead a survivor to develop homophobic feelings or to behave in a hyper-masculine way. Similarly, a female survivor may wish to hide her femininity by dressing or behaving in a masculine way to avoid sexual attention.

While there is a lack of robust evidence with regard to the impact of sexual violence on sexual orientation, many victims and survivors report being confused about their sexual orientation. For some survivors this confusion leads them to avoid any romantic relationships.

Beryl

Beryl was sexually abused by her older female cousin from the age of 11. This occurred whenever they had sleepovers or went on family vacations during school holidays. Beryl enjoyed being made to feel special and liked the sensations in her body when her cousin touched and stroked her intimately. As Beryl entered adulthood she became uncertain about her sexuality and found it excruciatingly difficult to date anyone. As a result she was unable to form any romantic attachment in her adult life.

For others the uncertainty is compounded by triggers associated with their abuse and what that evokes, rendering them fearful and doubtful of their sexual attraction or orientation, despite efforts to define their sexual identity.

Simon

From the age of five to nine Simon was raped by his older brother. As Simon entered adolescence he was sure that this had had no impact on his sexuality and he identified as heterosexual. His initial relationships with females were often complicated as he lacked relationship skills and was terrified of the SSA being exposed. In addition, he felt ashamed of his compulsion to watch pornography, especially gay porn. While this was arousing for him it was also extremely triggering as it brought back memories of being sexually abused by his older brother. This paralysed him to such an extent that he was unable to form romantic attachments or have sexual intimacy with either females or males.

The long-term effects of SSA can significantly impact on the sense of self and relationships, and lead to isolation and trauma-based loneliness. The fear of relationships can also affect professional relationships, making it hard to trust therapists and clinicians. The next chapter will explore how to work with survivors within a strengths-based, relational, trauma-informed practice approach which incorporates the Power Threat Meaning Framework and the importance of titrating exposure to traumatic experiences through a phased oriented model of treatment.

Further Reading

Boon, S., Steele, K., & van der Hart, O. (2011). *Coping with trauma-related dissociation: Skills training for patients and therapists*. W.W. Norton.

Caffaro, J.V., & Conn-Caffaro, A. (1998). *Sibling abuse trauma: Assessment and intervention strategies for children, families and adults*. Routledge.

Dell, P.F., & O'Neill, J.A. (2015). *Dissociation and the dissociative disorders: DSM-5 and beyond*. Routledge.

Fisher, J. (2017). *Healing the fragmented selves of trauma survivors*. Routledge.

Kezelman, C.A., & Stavropoulos, P.A. (2020). *Practice guidelines for identifying and treating complex trauma related dissociation*. Blue Knot Foundation.

McCartan, K., Anning, A., & Qureshi, E. (2021). *The impact of sibling sexual abuse on adults who were harmed as children*. UWE, Bristol Research Report.

Sanderson, C. (2013). *Counselling skills for working with trauma*. Jessica Kingsley Publishers.

Sanderson, C. (2015). *Responding to survivors of child sexual abuse: A pocket guide for professionals, partners, families and friends*. One in Four.

Sanderson, C. (2017). *Dissociation and dissociative disorders: Advice for adults suffering with dissociation and those working with them*. One in Four.

Sanderson, C. (2019). *Numbing the pain: A pocket guide for professionals supporting survivors of childhood sexual abuse and addiction*. One in Four.

Sanderson, C. (2022). *The warrior within: A One in Four handbook to aid recovery for survivors of childhood sexual abuse and violence* (4th edn). One in Four.

Steele, K., Boon, S., & Van der Hart, O. (2017). *Treating trauma related dissociation: A practical, integrative approach*. W.W. Norton.

van der Hart, O., Nijenhuis, E., & Steele, K. (2006). *The haunted self: Structural dissociation and the treatment of chronic traumatisation*. W.W. Norton.

Van der Kolk, B. (2015). *The body keeps the score: Mind, brain and body in the transformation of trauma*. Penguin Books.

CHAPTER 9

Working with Adult Survivors of Sibling Sexual Abuse: Trauma-Informed Practice

The complex nature of SSA can make it very difficult for survivors to legitimise their abuse and seek help as adults. Due to the confusion around the sexual experiences and shame, many survivors find it difficult to link the SSA to later difficulties in their lives. Repeated and systematic SSA, especially involving young children who are not able to understand or process what is happening, commonly results in dissociation and pushing the abuse elements of the experience out of conscious awareness.

This chapter will focus on how to manage the aftermath of SSA in adulthood, such as the impact of trauma and delayed trauma, the impact of disclosure and post-disclosure trauma, dissociation, emotional dysregulation, relationship difficulties, and compromised mental health. This is most effective when adopting a relational and strengths-based approach, which is lodged within a trauma-informed practice framework which includes an understanding of the Power Threat Meaning Framework (Johnstone & Boyle, 2018) and a phase-oriented approach to titrate exposure to the SSA experiences.

When working with adult survivors of SSA it is important that professionals and clinicians understand the complex nature of SSA and the difficulties around disclosure and legitimising the abuse. They will need to have an understanding of the nature of SSA, the impact of family dynamics, and recognise that some siblings who harm may also have been sexually abused and as such have 'dual status'. In addition, as many survivors minimise the experience and impact of SSA by viewing it as normative sexual experimentation, or a harmless game in which the sibling who has harmed is seen as a child who did not know what they were doing, practitioners need to be aware of delayed trauma. In addition, they need to ensure that they do not replicate previous professionals' minimisation of the SSA or dismissal of it as harmless (Sanderson, 2004).

Preparing to Work with Adult Survivors

To prepare for working with survivors of SSA it is necessary to gain as much knowledge as possible through specialist training and reading appropriate research. Ideally this would include a fuller understanding of trauma, the complex nature of sibling relationships, sexual development in children, and what is considered developmentally appropriate or inappropriate sexual behaviour in children, as well as the impact of SSA. Practitioners also need to be able to listen and talk about sex and sexual practices without embarrassment, shame, or arousal, as this will make it easier for survivors to talk about their experiences. In addition, practitioners will need to develop self-awareness about their own value system, and attitudes and beliefs around gender, power, the nature of sibling relationships, sexuality, and what constitutes abusive behaviour.

Along with specialist training, practitioners will need to commit to continuing professional development, as well as appropriate supervision, or specific case consultations. If working with a survivor triggers the practitioner's own childhood experiences, it is imperative that they seek support, and consider re-entering personal therapy to avoid projection or contamination of the client's material.

It is crucial that practitioners pace disclosure and not force this prematurely. This involves being mindful of the survivor's readiness to talk about shameful experiences that evoke confusing and unbearable feelings. When working with trauma it is also important to pace exposure to traumatic experiences to minimise the risk of re-traumatisation.

Barriers to Disclosure

There are countless barriers to disclosure which are in part due to survivors not being able to link what happened to them in childhood to its later impact. Many survivors of SSA report that in childhood they didn't feel any overt effects of the SSA and they only realised that it had a negative impact when entering intimate or sexual relationships in adulthood, or when entering therapy for entirely different presenting symptoms. Due to the confusing nature of SSA, survivors often do not recognise that there may be a link between SSA and later mental or physical health difficulties, relationship or sexual difficulties, or substance dependency.

Survivors who dissociated during their abuse will not have access to clear memories of the SSA and fear that their limited verbal recall will result in not being believed. This is compounded if there is a 'trauma bond' (Sanderson, 2013, 2022) which binds the siblings together. The switching between abusive and loving behaviour becomes the 'superglue that bonds' the relationship, which is so strong that anything which threatens that bond will be resisted.

To manage such cognitive dissonance, the survivor is compelled to seal off any negative beliefs about the abuser and to humanise rather than demonise them. In this the child compartmentalises the abuse components within the relationship while focusing on the positive and caring aspects. This necessitates 'thought blindness' in which reality is distorted to override the true nature of the relationship and normalise the abuser's behaviour. In focusing on the loving aspects of the sibling the child begins to see him or her as 'good' and the survivor as 'bad'. Over time the survivor develops an increasingly higher tolerance for abuse, which can become so entrenched that the survivor is unable to admit the abuse to self or others.

In addition, their crippling sense of shame and inability to trust makes it extremely difficult to explore their abuse experience with professionals until a degree of trust has been established. As a result SSA may not be disclosed during the early stages of therapy and only emerge when there is a degree of trust. While some survivors do allude to a history of SSA through coded messages, when these are not deciphered by the professional, it leaves them voiceless and unheard which impedes further exploration. This hinders the development of a secure and safe relationship in which to break the silence and secrecy.

Shame is a powerful silencer and the gatekeeper for anger and rage, especially if the survivor felt complicit in the abuse, or enjoyed the closeness with their sibling, or became sexually aroused. They typically feel ashamed of what happened and fear being re-shamed and stigmatised if the secret is exposed. Survivors also fear the consequences of disclosure such as the fragmentation of the family or splitting of loyalties, mandatory reporting, or being perceived as at risk of abusing their own children.

In order to facilitate disclosure, practitioners need to be open and engaged in bearing witness. They need to be able to convey empathy and compassion and demonstrate that they genuinely care. This is aided by sensitive pacing of the disclosure and psychological contact, and ensuring they do not rush the survivor, as this mimics the need to 'rush through' the abuse experience. Being present and in psychological contact with the survivor whether they are talking or silent is critical to demonstrate that they are heard rather than judged, rejected, or abandoned. It is also essential that practitioners are able to tolerate and validate the survivor's feelings, no matter how ambivalent, including feelings of love for the sibling who harmed them and how this links to a trauma bond (Sanderson, 2022).

It is critical to titrate exposure to the abuse experiences to minimise re-traumatisation. This is best done within a phase-oriented approach (Herman, 2001; Courtois & Ford, 2012; Sanderson, 2013, 2022; Baranowsky & Gentry, 2014; see Box 9.1). Gentle enquiry to encourage initial disclosure is often more helpful than direct questions which can be frightening and intrusive, and lead to traumatisation. While some survivors prefer being asked directly, others prefer a gentler approach.

If professionals feel uncomfortable about asking direct questions, it can help to develop a range of sensitive questions such as 'Has anyone done anything to you that you wish they hadn't?', 'Were there any things that happened in your childhood that confused or frightened you?', 'Has anyone ever made you feel special and then gone on to hurt you?', or 'Sometimes it is hard to talk about things that are confusing or frightening. I want you to know that the most important thing is for you to feel safe here, and that I am here for you if you want to talk and if you prefer not to' (Sanderson, 2019).

When the survivor does disclose a history of SSA it is essential to remember to ask questions about how they are now, and not just focus on memories and details of the abuse, as these can lead to numbing rather than making sense of the experiences. It is much more helpful to ask 'How do you feel the abuse has affected you?' or 'What did you have to do to survive?' or 'What sense did you make of the abuse?' and 'What would help you the most now?'

Practitioners will need to be respectful of the survivor's fear around disclosure and pace this sensitively to minimise the risk of post-disclosure trauma. They will also need to be aware of their own barriers in responding to disclosure of SSA such as disbelief, lack of knowledge or training, not knowing how to respond or facilitate disclosure, or opening Pandora's Box and making it worse for the survivor (Sanderson, 2016). Practitioners may also fear mandatory reporting, or litigation from the survivor's family or sibling, and shame around working with sexual violence (Sanderson, 2019).

It is also prudent for practitioners to be aware of their own attitudes to sex and sexuality (Sanderson, 2013) and to have knowledge about typical and atypical sexual development in children and have an understanding of sexually harmful behaviour in children (Sanderson, 2004, 2006).

Range of Therapeutic Modalities

There are a number of therapies that can be used when working with survivors of complex trauma which includes SSA. Current NICE guidelines advocate trauma focused cognitive behavioural therapy and eye movement desensitisation and reprocessing (EMDR). While EMDR has many treatment benefits for symptom reduction and the integration of processed traumatic material (Gelinas, 2003; Twombly, 2005; Steele & Van der Hart, 2009), it is best used within an overall treatment approach rather than as a standalone treatment. There are however risks of using EMDR with severely traumatised clients as premature exposure can reactivate traumatic memory too quickly (Gelinas, 2003; Twombly, 2005; Forgash & Knipe, 2008) and it is now considered to be most effective when employed within a phase-oriented approach to ensure a degree of stabilisation and a range of coping strategies to manage trauma symptoms and emotional self-regulation (Shapiro, 2009).

Cognitive-based therapies such as dialectical behavioural therapy, cognitive analytic therapy, and mindfulness-based stress reduction have also been found to be effective, as well as compassion focused therapy and acceptance and commitment therapy, which combine mindfulness with the practice of self-acceptance. Schema therapy can also be beneficial when working with personality adaptations and early schemas that emerge as a result of unmet needs in childhood.

Somatic therapies such as sensorimotor psychotherapy (Ogden, 2015) and Levine's somatic experiencing therapy (Levine, 1997; Payne et al., 2015) aim to modify trauma-related stress responses through bottom-up processing that directs attention to internal states through interoception, proprioception, and kinaesthesis. While these have considerable benefits when working with survivors of SSA, it is important to assess the readiness for these as many survivors find it too traumatising to be in their bodies and would benefit from trauma-safe adjustments (Sanderson, 2013, 2022; Rothschild, 2017).

Some survivors of SSA are unable to speak the unspeakable, and thus benefit more from non-verbal and bottom-up processing techniques to bridge the communication gap to what is split off and stored in the right brain. They may find expressive therapies such as any of the art and play therapies, or drama, dance, and movement therapies more accessible (Sanderson, 2022).

Survivors who are not ready to give voice to their experiences may find that their daily function is improved through other therapies such as animal assisted therapy, equine therapy, eco therapy, bibliotherapy, film therapy, or music therapy. Alternatively they can counterbalance the destructive elements of abuse through engaging in activities that are creative and constructive such as cooking, gardening, knitting, writing, or building as these are the antithesis of the destructive behaviours characteristic of SSA.

Whichever approach is used it is important that practitioners are aware that survivors of SSA are not homogeneous and there is no 'one-size-fits-all' approach. Survivors will vary with regard to preferred modalities depending on where they are in their process, their readiness to talk about their experiences, and what is most appealing and manageable for them. Survivors need to have the autonomy and choice to explore what is most helpful for them (Sanderson, 2022). Applying a trauma-informed practice and phase-oriented approach is generally considered to be the most effective approach for survivors of complex trauma and SSA (Herman, 2001; Courtois & Ford, 2012; Sanderson, 2013, 2022; Baranowsky & Gentry, 2014; Van der Kolk, 2015; Rothschild, 2017) as it acts as a scaffold to the practitioner's individual preferred modality.

Additionally, it is essential to have an understanding of the pervasive power and control dynamics in all forms of sexual violation including SSA, no matter how subtle or concealed. Survivors of SSA will have experienced a misuse of power and control, fear, excitement, and confusion which they could not process (Sanderson, 2013, 2022). To survive, survivors will have learnt to become compliant and submissive, and feel they have little or no choice or self-agency. To minimise the replication of the misuse of power and control, practitioners need to ensure that they provide a secure and safe therapeutic space in which trauma is seen through the eyes of each individual survivor, and ensure that power and control is equalised through promoting autonomy and choice. In encouraging survivors to be active agents in their recovery, the practitioner becomes a reliable and faithful companion on their journey to recovery (Sanderson, 2022).

The Power Threat Meaning Framework

To fully understand the impact of power and control on individuals it is important to view emotional distress and complex behaviours not just as symptoms but within the context of the person's experiences, and their attempts at making sense of these. The Power Threat Meaning Framework proposes an alternative to traditional models based on psychiatric diagnosis and its focus on symptoms (Johnstone & Boyle, 2018; Boyle & Johnstone, 2020). The emphasis in the framework is to understand 'what happened' to the person rather than 'what is wrong with' them. It is a way of understanding how people try to make sense of difficult and confusing experiences in order to gain meaning. Furthermore, it locates the emotional distress and concomitant behaviours as responses, or adaptations, to being controlled and the misuse of power. Practitioners need to ensure that they do not re-traumatise survivors by validating their narratives and link their responses to their abuse experiences rather than pathologising or shaming them for their 'symptoms'. By making the link between distress and the abuse of power survivors of SSA can begin to reduce shame and self-blame, and reclaim their power and control.

With this in mind practitioners need to structure their approach to encourage survivors to tell their story and focus on asking what has happened to them, how power was used to control them, and how this affected them. In addition, it is essential to explore what sense they made of their experiences and the meaning they have ascribed to these (Johnstone & Boyle, 2018; Boyle & Johnstone, 2020). Alongside this, practitioners need to help survivors to identify their threat responses and what they had to do to survive without judgement, and recognise which coping strategies are evoked in the present. This includes contextualising and understanding behaviours and responses that appear to be countertherapeutic as protective survival strategies rather than non-compliant, resistant, or avoidant. The focus needs to be on 'what happened to them' rather than 'what is wrong with them'.

Trauma-Informed Practice

The Power Threat Meaning Framework is aligned to the core principles of trauma-informed practice, namely those of safety, trustworthiness, collaboration, choice, and empowerment (Najavits, 2002; Elliott et al., 2005; Fallot & Harris, 2008; Butler et al., 2011; Quiros & Berger, 2015). Trauma-informed practice requires the ability to look at trauma through the eyes of each individual. The focus is on creating safety and trust through working collaboratively and promoting choices and respecting autonomy. It also identifies the individual's strengths and emphasises empowerment, that recovery from trauma is possible, and that there is hope (Fallot & Harris, 2008; Butler et al., 2011; Berger & Quiros, 2014; Quiros & Berger, 2015).

> Box 9.1 Fundamental principles of trauma-informed practice (adapted from Fallot & Harris, 2008; Quiros & Berger, 2015)
>
> 1. **Safety** – Both physical and emotional for the client. The physical environment, such as the location of the consulting room, placement of furniture etc., is crucial for the client to truly be and feel safe. Internal safety is achieved through amelioration of trauma symptoms and reduction in self-harming behaviours. Psychoeducation to increase awareness of the reactions to trauma and the impact of trauma symptoms
> 2. **Trustworthiness** – Trust is necessary for the therapeutic relationship, given the betrayal they have experienced. Trust must be built gradually by being clear and explicit with regard to the therapeutic process and a mutual respect for the practitioner and client responsibilities, as well as a mutual respect for the client's emotional limits and the practitioner's therapeutic capabilities
> 3. **Collaboration** – Collaboration between the client and the practitioner. The sharing of power becomes a vital tool and the client is seen as an expert in their lived experience. In essence, collaboration equalises the intrinsic power dynamics in the therapeutic process and promotes power in connection and mutuality
> 4. **Choice** – The principle of choice is activated by ensuring that

the client plays an active role in the planning and evaluation of treatment. This includes case formulation, therapeutic modality, as well as therapeutic goals, treatment, and outcome. The choice of type of intervention is essential to emphasise the client's rights and responsibilities
5. **Empowerment** – Recognising the resources, skills, and abilities that enabled the client to survive is crucial to ensure that they are not rendered powerless. The client's strengths and resilience need to be emphasised and cultivated to engender true empowerment

Survivors of SSA have learned that relationships are confusing and dangerous rather than a place of safety, and as such will be wary of entering the therapeutic relationship. It is crucial that practitioners create a secure base in which to foster internal and external safety in order for survivors to feel safe enough to reset their heightened alarm system by reducing subcortical activation and bring cortical functions such as cognition back online (Sanderson, 2013, 2022). In developing emotional self-regulation skills survivors will be able to feel more in control over their trauma symptoms.

In order to manage power dynamics ethically it is essential to reduce the intrinsic structural power in the therapeutic encounter by acknowledging and discussing power dynamics and the rights and responsibilities of both client and practitioner. This needs to be supported by a sharing of power and knowledge through psychoeducation and promoting equality, autonomy, agency, and choice. Alongside sharing power, practitioners must be able to modulate control dynamics by encouraging survivors to take control in their lives as well as in the therapeutic space, and be willing to relinquish control by not being too directive or expecting the survivor to work at a pace that is unmanageable for them. In addition, it is important to acknowledge that the therapist is not the only source of healing and to encourage the survivor to seek other sources of support such as a survivor group.

Due to the sense of betrayal by people who appear to be trustworthy, it is critical that practitioners are experienced as trustworthy, and that this is conveyed to, as well as felt by, the survivor. Survivors of SSA commonly find it difficult to trust, and practitioners need to consistently demonstrate their trustworthiness through honesty and authenticity, and reduce the need for mind reading. As sexual abuse is predicated on deception and betrayal, survivors are hyper-vigilant to any cues that herald danger or threat. To ensure that they do not replicate abuse dynamics around authenticity or clarity, practitioners need to be explicit in terms of boundaries, managing expectations, articulating therapist and client responsibilities, and respecting clients' emotional limits and not judging them when they feel overwhelmed, stuck, or unable to fully engage in the work. They need to ensure that they do not shame survivors by interpreting their behaviour as resistant when in essence these are protective survival strategies that have been activated as a result of fear or shame (Sanderson, 2013, 2022).

Practitioners will need to be patient as it takes time to build trust, with some survivors never able to trust fully. The lack of trust in others is exacerbated by the doubt and lack of trust in themselves which also needs to be explored. Many survivors find that as they begin to trust in themselves they find it easier to trust others. It is advisable not to force or push trust but allow it to evolve over time. This is best facilitated through a dyadic process in which the therapist needs to trust the survivor to enable him or her to trust themselves, as well as conveying their trustworthiness through honesty and authenticity.

Some survivors search for evidence of trustworthiness through testing behaviours and therapists need to understand these as survival strategies to regulate closeness rather than non-compliance, or personalise any criticism or undermining of competency or care. Survivors will benefit from a calm, contained, and consistent response that frames such tests as a protective survival strategy for the perceived threat of trusting, in case they are taken advantage of, hurt, or rejected.

The building of trust is also aided through psychoeducation by providing non-biased information about trauma symptoms, the impact of these, and the dynamics of the therapeutic process. This psychoeducation and openness to talk about the nature of the therapeutic relationship, and challenges around trust, as well as traumatic transference and counter transference, are crucial to developing trust in the therapeutic alliance. Therapists will need to be honest and authentic as they demonstrate their capacity to bear witness without judgement and show fortitude in the presence of unspeakable experiences, wordless terror, and unbearable feelings.

Dionne

Dionne had been sexually abused by her older brother, and although she told her parents they did not believe her; the abuse continued until she left home aged 16. She was extremely wary of her therapist and found it hard to allow herself to connect with them. In exploring this she recognised that she was unable to trust anyone, not her family, her friends, or partners. In exploring how this played out she described that she would consistently set tests for anyone who tried to get close to her. This would take the form of her ignoring their attempts to connect, not returning telephone calls or texts, cancelling prearranged meetings at the last minute, or just not turning up, and at times being rude or hostile. This was often because she didn't feel safe and needed to control the degree of attachment.

The building of the therapeutic relationship was slow and painstaking, with a lot of 'approach and avoid' behaviour.

As Dionne began to invest in the therapeutic relationship, she began to test whether she could truly trust her therapist. This initially manifested as consistently coming late to sessions, or not turning up at all. When she did come she would avoid talking about what had happened and often delayed payment. Attempts to explore this were extremely painful for Dionne as it put her in contact with the myriad betrayals in childhood. Every time there seemed to be some progress, Dionne would leave voicemail messages in between sessions berating her therapist for the slowness of the therapeutic work, undermining competency and doubting the genuineness of her therapist's care.

As she identified the triggers that activated testing behaviours, it emerged that Dionne also found it hard to trust herself. Realising this, the focus of the work shifted to developing trust in herself, her perception, and her experiences, which enabled Dionne to reclaim her reality and reduce her pervasive self-doubt, supported by her therapist's belief in her. As she began to trust herself she began to trust her therapist without needing to test them and they were able to build the therapeutic relationship based on mutual trust.

To ensure that survivors feel safe practitioners need to promote choices especially when working with survivors of SSA who were not given choices during their abuse, or were blamed for their participation. It is essential to provide as much as choice as possible in the therapeutic setting such as where to sit, the positioning of the chairs, and the proximity and physical space between practitioner and client. Survivors need to be able to see the exit door, and reach it easily. They also need to feel that they have a choice in how closely the chairs are positioned, and at which angle.

Many survivors feel uncomfortable sitting directly opposite the practitioner as this elicits shame, and feel more comfortable if the chairs are placed at an angle, or side by side, at least initially. This also helps to regulate eye contact as it is often under the gaze of others that shame is induced and trauma-wise practitioners (TWP) need to be mindful that the intensity of eye gaze and eye contact can be triggering and lead to dissociation (Sanderson, 2013, 2015). Practitioners are encouraged to share the regulation of eye gaze and proximity with each individual client to find the optimal distance that feels safe for them. It is helpful at the beginning of each session to check with the client how comfortable they feel and to spend a few minutes settling into the therapeutic space through breathing and grounding skills.

Sharon

Whenever Sharon entered the consulting room her head was bent and her eyes lowered as she shrank back into her chair. It was clear that she was terrified and that being in the therapeutic space activated her fear response. Her therapist suggested she take a moment to settle into the room. Once she looked a little less terrified the therapist checked with her how she felt about the positioning of the chairs and if it would help to increase or decrease the proximity so she would find the optimal space between them. To experiment the therapist gently moved their chair while checking Sharon's body language and asked her how this felt. After several attempts they found the space most comfortable for Sharon. After settling into the space the therapist checked with Sharon about how she felt about being looked at by them; Sharon replied that she found that hard as she felt scrutinised and ashamed. She began to realise that she often felt this when in relationships as it reminded her of when her brother would stare at her intensely. The therapist suggested they experiment with eye gaze so it didn't feel too intrusive. Sharon felt most comfortable if she didn't look directly at the eyes and directed the therapist's gaze to a slightly lower part of her face. They also experimented with the positioning of the chairs, and moving them so the therapist was at a slight angle, where Sharon felt less scrutinised. Gradually over time as she felt less ashamed Sharon was able to look at the therapist and they were able to have more sustained eye-to-eye contact.

In addition, survivors need to feel that they have a choice in whether to talk or not to talk, and to regulate silence. While therapeutic silences can be fruitful opportunities to reflect and access feelings, for many survivors silence is experienced as punitive and is reminiscent of the abuse. It is essential that practitioners regulate the silence appropriately, and that prolonged silences do not trigger or activate shame or dissociative states. The shame associated with SSA is easily evoked in prolonged silence, and survivors may interpret this as shaming or rejecting. Practitioners also need to distinguish between therapeutic silences and silence that occurs due to unspeakable terror or dissociation.

> ### Jack
> 25-year-old Jack who had been sexually abused by his older sister from the age of eight would often become silent in sessions with his therapist. This would invariably be induced when he tried to remember the details of what happened to him. He would often look terrified and would try to mouth what he wanted to say with no sound, which exacerbated his terror and shame. In these moments his therapist would modulate their tone of voice to gently reassure him that he was safe. This would help to regulate his hypo-aroused state and enabled him to regain a sense of calm. At other times Jack's eyes glazed over while his facial features were bereft of any emotions. As he entered a dissociative state, Jack would become unresponsive and unreachable. In order to bring him back into the present his therapist again would modulate their tone of voice by being steadier and more instructional, using his name and asking him to look at them. This would be accompanied with placing one end of a scarf on his hand for him to hold while his therapist held the other end so that he felt tethered and connected, and safe to return to the present.

Throughout the therapeutic process and journey to recovery survivors must be encouraged to make autonomous choices and have these respected and supported by the practitioner. This is not always easy as some survivors find it hard to make choices as they believe they have been stripped of their self-agency and doubt themselves in making any decision. Practitioners also need to acknowledge that clients from diverse cultures will have different expectations with regard to therapy and the therapeutic relationship, and prefer to see the therapist as expert and elevate their status as this makes them feel safer.

Rukshana

Rukshana found therapy extremely difficult as she felt it challenged the values and beliefs that had been inculcated throughout her life that as a female she had no voice, she should respect her elders, and comply with whatever males decided for her. This rendered her vulnerable to her sexual abuse by her older brother and cousin. She felt that she could not challenge the abuse and that she had no choice other than to comply.

Rukshana was confused when her therapist asked what she would like to achieve through therapy and how they might work together to attain her desired goals. She would say she didn't know and that it was her therapist's job to decide for her as they were the expert. Never having been given any self-agency she had no idea how to acquire this, and it was frightening to even contemplate it.

Rukshana was also terrified of making any decision in case it was the wrong one. When she and her therapist explored this, Rukshana described that she felt that the sexual abuse was her fault because she wanted to go and visit her cousin and persuaded her brother to take her to his house. This decision she believed led to her abuse, and her shame and guilt led her to doubt herself whenever faced with a decision. It was safer not to make any decisions and not to express her desires or needs. During the work, her therapist would encourage her to find ways of identifying and then expressing her needs, and hypothesise how these might be met. As she became more confident in expressing her needs in session, her therapist encouraged her to express how these could best be met. Rukshana would practise these in the safety of the session until she felt more confident to express these to trusted others. Making that decision, being heard, and appropriately responded to enabled her to start making decisions and claim the self-agency she had been denied. While this was not easy as it caused conflict in the family, over time Rukshana was able to reduce her self-doubt and believe in herself, and in reducing the self-doubt was more able to challenge and express her needs. As the therapy progressed, she was able to identify and challenge her therapist with regard to some of their reflections and hypotheses, and make her own choices and decisions, including when she was ready to end therapy.

To equalise power it is helpful for practitioners to adopt a collaborative and non-hierarchical approach in which survivors are encouraged to take an active role in their healing and empowerment. To facilitate this therapists need to ensure that the therapeutic relationship is co-created and based on mutuality (Miller, 2015; Jordan, 2017). In being explicit and transparent therapists reduce the need of the survivor to 'mind read', and promote self-agency in a safe way.

Alongside collaboration, TWPs need to ensure they respect the survivor's right to make autonomous choices such as the chosen treatment modality, case formulation, intervention, planning, and the evaluation of treatment. This will enable them to restore control and build trust in their self-agency as well as making life choices post therapy.

Equalising and sharing of power is crucial to facilitate empowerment in which the survivor is accorded respect and seen as expert in their own life and experiences. Most importantly practitioners need to recognise and validate the resources and skills that the survivor already has which have enabled them to survive such as courage and resilience. In focusing on their strengths, survivors will feel empowered rather than rendered helpless. This can lay the foundation for further empowerment through the cultivation and acquisition of more skills and reclaiming control over their bodies and restoring reality. This is hard to achieve with some survivors, who are afraid of their power in case they abuse it as their sibling did. It is important that practitioners explore this and remind them power comes with responsibility to do no harm, rather than the abuse of power.

The Phase-Oriented Approach to Working with Trauma

Whichever type of treatment option is accessed, it is important that it is regulated and sensitively paced so that the survivor is not re-traumatised. This is best achieved through a phase-oriented model using the principles of trauma-informed practice, which can either be used as a single specialist approach or be incorporated into an existing or preferred treatment approach (Herman, 2001; Courtois & Ford, 2012; Sanderson, 2013, 2022; Baranowsky & Gentry, 2014). The advantage of a phased approach is that it is flexible and survivors can go at their own pace to build the necessary resources to enable them to explore the trauma without becoming re-traumatised, and acquire skills that will promote resilience and post-traumatic growth (Ford et al., 2005; Courtois & Ford, 2012; Van der Kolk, 2015; Rothschild, 2017, 2021; Sanderson, 2022).

While the model consists of three distinct phases – **Stabilisation**, **Processing**, and **Integration** – practitioners need to be aware that the phases are dynamic and not linear, and that there is considerable fluidity and oscillation between phases. This is especially the case in high-functioning survivors who may have disavowed the SSA through causing a split in self-states characteristic of structural dissociation in which one part of the personality has disavowed all traumatic experiences while another part is immersed in trauma. Such survivors may present with delayed trauma which only emerges in therapy when exploring their childhood experiences in more detail.

It is important to note that Judith Herman in her latest book, *Truth and Repair* (Herman, 2023), has added a fourth phase to aid recovery, which she calls Justice (see Table 9.1). In this stage Herman argues that in order for survivors to fully heal they need to have some degree of justice from the larger community, which includes not just the perpetrator(s) but all those who have been complicit in the abuse, such as passive or indifferent bystanders, institutions, the criminal justice system, and wider communities and society who often blame the victim.

Emily

Emily, 33, a highly successful consultant, entered therapy due to a history of depression and relationship difficulties. She was always elegantly dressed, exuded poise, and was extremely articulate, which belied her longstanding diagnosis of depression. Emily was able to give a seemingly clear account of her life and reported that she had a happy childhood with no ACEs, and no history of trauma. In exploring what she hoped to achieve through therapy and in assessing her readiness for therapy, her therapist believed that she was ready to proceed. Several months into the therapeutic work Emily started to explore her relationship with her siblings. While she described these as generally good, her demeanour would change when talking about her step-brother, who moved into the family home when she was three years old. He was very affectionate, paid her a lot of attention, and was happy to play the games she wanted to. Liam would often want to play doctors which involved him examining her intimately. This was confusing as sometimes it felt nice and other times uncomfortable when he would insert things into her vagina. When she told Liam that she felt confused he said that this is the sort of game all sisters and brothers played. As he was never violent towards her she felt that this was normal and harmless.

As Emily explored these experiences in more detail she would begin to lose her voice and become unresponsive. She would stare into the distance and become unreachable for considerable periods of time. When she was able to come back into the present moment she would blink her eyes and look at her therapist in a puzzled way as though she did not know who they were. It was clear that whenever she spoke about Liam, she would go into a dissociative state which suggested that he was associated with unbearable and overwhelming feelings and sensations. This suggested that she was switching between self-states characteristic of structural dissociation as she would have no recollection of having 'zoned out' and not recognising her therapist when coming back into the present.

Given these dissociative symptoms it was necessary for her therapist to pause exploration of the SSA she experienced and to focus on phase one work to find ways to manage her dissociative symptoms. This was crucial to ensure that Emily could acquire the skills to regulate her feelings around her step-brother, integrate the two self-states, and develop distress tolerance, before any further exploration of the SSA.

All four phases are inter-related and inter-dependent and equally important as each phase builds on the gains and skills mastered in previous phases. It is worth noting that severely traumatised survivors may not be able to progress beyond phase one. This should not be interpreted as failure as recovery is not dependent on remembering. What is essential is to be emotionally regulated and be able to live in the present rather than be catapulted back into the past (Van der Kolk, 2015).

The length of time for each phase is not measured in terms of time, but rather in the mastery of skills acquired and cultivated at each phase. Rather than focus on the SSA prematurely, the aim is to create a safe and secure base in which to build internal and external safety and enable the survivor to restore control over trauma symptoms through affect regulation using grounding skills to build distress tolerance before remembering and processing SSA experiences.

This is accompanied by psychoeducation in order to understand the impact of SSA and to normalise trauma symptoms as adaptations and reactions to threat which enabled them to survive. Psychoeducation enables survivors to recognise that trauma resets the emotional alarm system on either high alert resulting in hyper-arousal and hyper-vigilance or shut down as seen in hypo-arousal (Sanderson, 2016, 2022). When hyper-aroused, subcortical areas of the brain such as the amygdala predominate, or come online, while the cortical areas of the brain involved with cognition, thinking, and decision making are reduced, and go offline. In contrast in hypo-arousal all systems shut down.

In order to process the SSA and concomitant overwhelming feelings, survivors need to feel safe to acquire the requisite skills to gain mastery over trauma symptoms and to mute or deactivate the subcortical areas of the brain involved in threat responses, so that the cortical areas of the brain can come back online.

As the phases are not measured in time but on the acquisition and mastery of skills, it is critical that practitioners assess readiness to move on to the next phase, and be prepared to move back and forth fluidly (Cloitre et al., 2012; Courtois & Ford, 2012). It is essential to remember that oscillation between phases is not an indicator of failure, but rather an opportunity to reinforce skills and consolidate gains made. Newly acquired skills and strategies may need to be repeated numerous times before they are fully consolidated to enable emotions and cognitions to be processed and integrated.

Table 9.1 Phase-oriented approach when working with adult survivors (adapted from Herman, 2015, 2023)

Phase one: Stabilisation	Phase two: Processing	Phase three: Integration	Phase four: Justice
Safety – internal and external	Process trauma experiences	Integrate the abuse experiences	Justice from the larger community, including perpetrator(s), indifferent bystanders, institutions, the criminal justice system, and wider communities
Identify resources and cultivate these	Realisation of harm done	Create meaning	
Psychoeducation	Restore reality	Reconnect to self, others, and the world	
Grounding skills – breathing, mindfulness	Challenge distorted perceptions	Build resilience	
Build the therapeutic relationship	Reallocate shame	Post-traumatic growth	
	Grieve losses		Public recognition of harm done, accountability, and responsibility

Phase One: Stabilisation

In phase one the focus is on creating safety, promoting self-care, improving daily life, identifying the survivor's strengths and coping strategies, including the adaptive components of dissociation, and assessing their current needs. This needs to include a risk assessment if the harming sibling still exerts power and control over the survivor. During this phase emphasis is placed on developing stabilisation skills such as grounding and emotional self-regulation in order to manage overwhelming trauma reactions, and building a personalised recovery toolkit (Sanderson, 2019, 2022).

In order to restore control over trauma reactions and reset the alarm system, it is important to identify the range of triggers that lead to emotional dysregulation. Initially, this involves recognising and identifying emotions, and developing grounding techniques such as breathing, mindfulness, and self-soothing skills that increase distress tolerance and widen the window of tolerance (Ogden et al., 2006) by regulating overwhelming trauma reactions. These techniques can include regular exercise to discharge trapped energy, adrenaline, and distress hormones (Levine, 1997; Payne et al., 2015) or relaxation and mindfulness skills that pay attention to body sensations and increase physical awareness (Van der Kolk, 2015; Rothschild, 2017).

Rather than meditation or relaxation techniques that involve closing of the eyes, which is likely to trigger the alarm system and activate dissociation, it is better to start off with muscle clenching and progressive muscular relaxation. This involves the tensing and relaxing of various muscle groups to allow the survivor to feel more in control over their body rather than entering a dissociative state. Similarly, mindfulness can impact negatively on some survivors and needs to incorporate trauma-safe adjustments such as shorter exposure, open eyes, and combining interoception with proprioception (Rothschild, 2017, 2021; Van der Hart & Rydberg, 2019; Sanderson, 2022).

Survivors whose default setting is dissociation, and who find it difficult to remain present despite their arsenal of stabilisation skills, can be helped to stay in the present by making notes in session as they are likely to forget the content of the session if they have dissociated. This has a dual purpose in keeping hands busy which reduces the dissociation and keeping a record of what was explored in session. Some survivors may wish to record sessions to remind them what was discussed, or appreciate a short written summary from the practitioner.

Aaron

Aaron was highly dissociative as a result of severe SSA in early childhood committed by his two older brothers who would take it in turns to rape him. Despite exploring a number of techniques to manage the dissociation in session, Aaron found that sometimes he would zone out and not remember what he and the therapist had spoken about. One technique he found helpful to stay present was for him to hold one end of a scarf and his therapist to hold the other end, and for them each to twist their respective ends, a bit like wringing a towel. This helped Aaron to stay connected with his therapist and stay in the present. However, he often reported that, while it helped the more pronounced dissociative episodes, he often still felt fuzzy in session, and invariably uncertain about what was explored afterwards. His therapist suggested that Aaron take notes as they talked, as this would enable him to remain focused and gave him a contemporaneous record of the session. Aaron found this extremely useful as it reduced his feelings of unreality and uncertainty and provided a clearer record of what was happening in therapy. In addition, it was agreed that the therapist would summarise the previous session at the beginning of each session so that he could compare notes and help orientate Aaron for the forthcoming session. Aaron immediately felt safer and more grounded and less apprehensive about his sessions.

Learning new skills for emotional self-regulation to help the survivor stay in their window of tolerance is best achieved through consistent practice. It is helpful to build relaxation and distress tolerance techniques into every session especially at the beginning of the session and before leaving. The most important thing is to help the survivor experiment with a mixture of techniques rather than prescribing a single one. This will allow them to discover the techniques that work best for them, so that they are more able to regulate their emotions.

Psychoeducation is crucial in understanding how the body reacts to distress and to make sense of how trauma impacts on the mind and body. It also helps the survivor to make the link between SSA, trauma symptoms, and emotional dysregulation. This, alongside the stabilisation skills, will enable them to learn more adaptive skills to regulate their emotional reactions and tolerate distress when exploring memories of SSA.

Reframing symptoms as adaptations to threat and confusion, or as survival strategies, allows the survivor to have a better understanding of their behaviours. Psychoeducation also empowers the survivor to regain a sense of control and reduce shame and self-blame thereby allowing them to develop compassion for the self and what has happened to them.

Some of the components in the stabilisation phase, such as psychoeducation and grounding skills, can be delivered as group workshops, from which survivors can progress into one-to-one sessions. Many survivors report that group work which emphasises raising awareness and understanding SSA is an invaluable source of support that helps them make sense of their abuse experiences and the link to addiction (Sanderson, 2019).

Phase Two: Processing
Once the survivor has mastered stabilisation skills and widened their window of tolerance, they can enter phase two which focuses on processing the SSA experiences, flashbacks, and intrusive memories. In processing their experiences, survivors can come to realise the harm done and become aware of distorted perceptions of self, others, and the world which can be challenged to restore reality and belief in themselves. In addition, survivors can begin to reallocate shame and responsibility, and grieve the many losses associated with SSA. In releasing the pain and sorrow, they can begin to feel empathy and self-compassion for the child that was hurt and betrayed.

Remembering and realisation can be excruciatingly painful, especially if the survivor has dissociated from the experiences, or buried them. Practitioners must make sure that this exploration is appropriately paced so that the survivor is neither rushed nor becomes too focused on recovering memories and details of the abuse, as these may lead to desensitisation and numbing rather than integration. As feelings and memories are revived it is important to help the survivor to grieve their losses and begin to make meaning of their SSA.

Practitioners also need to recognise that remembering is not the road to recovery and healing (Van der Kolk, 2015) and that some survivors do not need to remember, or process every detail of the abuse experience. Many survivors can live satisfying lives without having remembered every aspect of their childhood experiences. The focus needs to be on helping the survivor to regain control over their trauma symptoms so that they are not catapulted back into the trauma or become plagued by intrusive memories, flashbacks, or nightmares (Sanderson, 2022). The amount of processing needs to be balanced by the client's needs and the extent to which unprocessed material is haunting them and impeding their everyday life, combined with the practitioner's assessment and observations, rather than being enforced by rigid expectations on either side.

Phase Three: Integration

The final phase aims to integrate the abuse experiences and create meaning. This paves the way for post-traumatic growth, in which the survivor is able to reconnect to the self, others, and the world. As their view of themselves and others changes, they can form healthy attachments to others without fear or shame, and begin to live in the present (Sanderson, 2019, 2022). The renewed energy and vitality prompts many survivors to reclaim their lives and to live their lives more fully, including making more empowered choices about their purpose in life, with regard to career choices and retraining. In essence, post-traumatic growth allows for renewed purpose and meaning, a greater appreciation of life, vitality, as well as feeling more alive. This can be a transformative process for both survivor and practitioner as it highlights the resilience of the human spirit.

As interpersonal trauma and SSA impacts on attachment and relationships it is essential to combine the trauma-informed practice model with a strengths-based relational approach which emphasises the centrality of the therapeutic relationship. The healing power of the therapeutic relationship is explored in the following chapter along with how this can restore relational worth and provide a safe space to build relationship skills.

Phase Four: Justice

This phase is predicated on Herman's (2023) proposition that for survivors to fully heal they need to have some degree of justice from the larger community: the perpetrator(s), those who have been complicit in the abuse such as passive or indifferent bystanders, institutions, the criminal justice system, and wider communities and society who often blame the victim. Survivors need acknowledgement of the harm that has been done and the impact of secondary traumatisation through stigmatisation – not being believed and not wishing to bear witness – to fully heal. According to Herman, this necessitates a public recognition of the wrongdoing, harm, and suffering inherent in sexual violence and abuse. This along with the accountability, responsibility, and compassion for those who have been harmed reduces blame, marginalisation, and stigmatisation and is a powerful way to promote cultural change in which 'injury to one, is injury to all' (Herman, 2023), and paves the path to justice for all.

Further Reading

Baranowsky, A., & Gentry, J.E. (2014). *Trauma practice: Tools for stabilization and recovery*. Hogrefe Publishing.

Boyle, M., & Johnstone, L. (2020). *A straight talking introduction to the Power Threat Meaning Framework: An alternative to psychiatric diagnosis*. PCCS Books.

Butler, L.D., Critelli, F.M., & Rinfrette, E.S. (2011). Trauma-informed care and mental health. *Directions in Psychiatry, 31*(3), 197–212.

Cloitre, M., Courtois, C.A., Ford, J.D., Green, B.L., Alexander, P., Briere, J., & Van der Hart, O. (2012). The ISTSS expert consensus treatment guidelines for complex PTSD in adults. ISTSS. https://istss.org/ISTSS_Main/media/Documents/ComplexPTSD.pdf

Courtois, C.A., & Ford, J.D. (2012). *Treatment of complex trauma: A sequenced, relationship-based approach*. Guilford Press.

Herman, J.L. (2001). *Trauma and recovery* (2nd edn). Basic Books.

Herman, J.L. (2023). *Truth and repair: How trauma survivors envision justice*. Basic Books.

Johnstone, L., & Boyle, M. with Cromby, J., Dillon, J., Harper, D., Kinderman, P., Longden, E., Pilgrim, D., & Read, J. (2018). *The Power Threat Meaning Framework: Towards the identification of patterns in emotional distress, unusual experiences and troubled or troubling behaviour, as an alternative to functional psychiatric diagnosis*. British Psychological Society.

Levine, P.A. (1997). *Waking the tiger*. North Atlantic Books.

Quiros, L., & Berger, R. (2015). Responding to the socio-political complexity of trauma: An integration of theory and practice. *Journal of Loss and Trauma, 20*(2), 149–159.

Rothschild, B. (2000). *The body remembers: The psychophysiology of trauma and trauma treatment*. W.W. Norton.

Rothschild, B. (2017). *The body remembers. Volume 2: Revolutionizing trauma treatment*. W.W. Norton.

Sanderson, C. (2006). *Counselling adult survivors of child sexual abuse* (3rd edn). Jessica Kingsley Publishers.

Sanderson, C. (2013). *Counselling skills for working with trauma*. Jessica Kingsley Publishers.

Sanderson, C. (2015). *Counselling skills for working with shame*. Jessica Kingsley Publishers.

Sanderson, C. (2022). *The warrior within: A One in Four handbook to aid recovery for survivors of childhood sexual abuse and violence* (4th edn). One in Four.

Van der Kolk, B. (2015). *The body keeps the score: Mind, brain and body in the transformation of trauma*. Penguin Books.

CHAPTER 10

Working with Adult Survivors of Sibling Sexual Abuse: The Therapeutic Relationship

This chapter will highlight the power of the healing relationship and its role in building trust, restoring relational worth, and developing relationship skills. It is through the therapeutic relationship that survivors are able to reconnect to self and others, and build healthy relationships. The chapter also explores the myriad challenges of working with survivors of SSA such as vicarious traumatisation and compassion fatigue, and the importance of practitioner self-care to minimise the risk of burnout and secondary traumatic stress.

The therapeutic relationship is fundamental to restore relational worth and aid recovery. Practitioners will need to honour the survivor's willingness to trust you despite repeated betrayal, as this indicates that hope is not extinguished and signals an opportunity to transform the dehumanisation of abuse through a human relationship. It is also an opportunity for the survivor to experience new ways of relating and relationship skills which they can use to build or rebuild relationships with others, including family members. To undo the effects of SSA, it is crucial that practitioners are able to offer a genuinely warm, human relationship in which the survivor is valued and respected. To achieve this it is crucial to adopt a collaborative and non-hierarchical approach in which the survivor is able to take equal control of their healing rather than being controlled and directed by the therapist and their therapeutic modality (Sanderson, 2013).

Practitioners need to be emotionally available and attuned to the survivor and be fully engaged, as a detached, blank screen approach is often experienced as re-traumatising. The emphasis needs to be on being able to 'be with' the survivor rather than 'doing to them'. This is vital to create a collaborative working alliance in which shared agreements are made about expectations of both parties, and how these can be managed, along with relational safety, especially as the therapeutic relationship unfolds and grows. Alongside this, practitioners need to be clear and explicit in their communication to reduce the need to 'mind read'. Survivors have learned to mind read in order to protect themselves, and in the presence of unclear or mixed messages will do so in the therapeutic relationship. Practitioners need to regularly check the quality of the communication in terms of what is said, received, and how that is interpreted.

Practitioners will need to be able to relinquish control at times, be non-directive, be non-coercive, flexible, and pace the work within limits that are manageable for the survivor (Sanderson, 2019). This necessitates establishing a supportive, non-judgemental, non-shaming, and sensitively attuned therapeutic relationship in which the survivor feels safe.

While working with survivors can be extremely tough and demanding, it is also the most rewarding work. It can be life changing for both the survivor and practitioner.

Creating a Secure Base

In order to work most effectively with survivors of SSA it is crucial to establish a safe, secure setting in which the survivor can pace their recovery. It is critical that the work is not rushed, as this is reminiscent of the abuse. It is more effective to pace the work that is manageable for the survivor so they can feel more in control of the work. The therapeutic relationship needs to be human, and based on genuine care and warmth and mutual respect for the client's knowledge of their lived experience. To equalise power and control dynamics, practitioners are cautioned not to make assumptions and to offer reflections and thoughts as possibilities or hypotheses rather than prescriptive interpretations which can invalidate the survivor's experiences (Cozolino, 2021).

It is also important to provide choices and not pressurise survivors to comply with what the practitioner thinks is right. While practitioners' intuitions are a rich source for ideas they are not the only way of healing. It is important to acknowledge that this is the survivor's process and that the therapist is merely accompanying him or her on their journey. To minimise the risk of confusion, distortion of reality, and to reduce the need to mind read it is important to be explicit rather than leave things to interpretation. It is also crucial that practitioners recognise their limitations and do not over-promise.

As the healing process is not linear it is essential to be patient when survivors become distracted, or diverted, or stuck, and not misinterpret this as resistance. Survivors find it extremely difficult to trust and they will need to test to what extent they can trust the therapist. Practitioners need to be mindful that trust is built over time and insisting on trust too early can put unnecessary pressure on the survivor and impede the therapeutic relationship.

In addition, it is vital to create a collaborative working alliance in which shared agreements are made about expectations of both parties, and how these can be managed, along with relational safety, especially as the therapeutic relationship unfolds and grows. In order for the therapeutic process to be truly empowering, agreements need to be bidirectional rather than imposed and controlled by either party, and be open to negotiation as the therapeutic relationship evolves. This is essential at a very fundamental level such as the proximity of the chairs and eye gaze. Giving survivors a choice in this conveys respect for their personal space and demonstrates that they have a choice in creating safety in therapeutic space.

It is also prudent to have regular reviews of how the survivor feels about the therapeutic process, the regulation of connection, the therapeutic goals, and to what extent these are being achieved. Through regular open discussion both the survivor and practitioner can stay on track and revise and re-negotiate as necessary (Sanderson, 2022) to more effectively manage both client and practitioner expectations, and retain a realistic, positive, and hopeful outcome.

Bearing in mind that survivors tend to experience relationships as sources of danger rather than comfort, practitioners need to be mindful when building the therapeutic relationship that the attachment system will be activated which, rather than induce a sense of comfort and safety, can engender anxiety, fear, and dissociation. As proximity and intimacy can lead to the hyper-activation of the attachment system it has the potential to trigger frightening material, flashbacks, and intrusive memories.

Given the fears around being connected and the oscillation between wanting to be connected and pulling away, it is helpful to check with the survivor how connected they feel during sessions, and especially when there is an energetic shift in the therapeutic space. This can be effected by having a scale of 1–5 with 1 feeling disconnected and 5 feeling connected, and checking with the client where they are on the scale at various moments in the session, either at the beginning or the end, or when they have been triggered by something, or there has been a rupture or an impasse. It can also help for the practitioner to state the degree of connection they feel if appropriate and to explore any shifts between the survivor and the practitioners. In addition, it enables both to identify triggers which deactivate the connection, and explore ways of reconnecting.

This can be done by rewinding to what the survivor was feeling or experiencing immediately prior to the disconnection and explore what is needed to restore the connection. Another helpful technique is to use a ball of wool with the survivor holding one end and the practitioner holding the other end. This acts as a physical representation of a thread that connects survivor and practitioner. You can also experiment with the tension of the wool and see how it feels when there is a strong connection and when the connection is weaker.

Mable

Mable entered therapy in her late 40s. She was single and had never been in a romantic or sexual relationship. Having been sexually abused by her older sister throughout much of her childhood, she was confused about her sexuality and feared closeness and connection with others and felt safer being on her own. Initially Mable was very reserved and overly contained with restricted body movement. She would rarely show any affect, or changes in facial expression or body language. As she and her therapist explored her SSA and its impact it was clear that Mable was terrified of people as she feared being hurt and shamed for her part in the SSA. She described how, although she knew what her sister was doing to her was wrong, it made her feel special, and some of the sexual activity felt nice and gave her pleasure, so much so that when her sister left home she felt bereft.

In exploring her history of SSA and its impact Mable reported that she found relationships with both males and females incredibly difficult and had not had any close friendships in either childhood or adulthood, and that whenever people attempted to get close to her she would become hostile and treat them badly. She had also not been able to form any romantic relationships as she was unsure of her sexuality and did not want to risk being sexually close to anyone.

It became clear to her therapist that Mable yearned to be connected to and in relationship with someone, but she was also terrified of this and needed to keep people at bay. This was evident in the therapeutic relationship as she would reach out and connect with her therapist, then retreat and avoid any psychological contact. This was often accompanied by anger and hostility, especially when she felt ashamed. To help increase awareness of her sense of connectedness and triggers that deactivated connection, Mable was encouraged to rewind to what was happening for her prior to the energetic shift, and explore that to understand the triggers that led to her to retreat. To preserve the connection between her and her therapist Mable found the use of the ball of wool exercise particularly helpful as she could see that she could be connected even if she couldn't permit herself to feel it. This enabled Mable to allow herself to internalise the connection and explore her feelings of both the terror of feeling connected and the hurt of feeling disconnected in a safer way. In pacing this, Mable was gradually able to remain more connected without retreating, and as she internalised this, the need for the ball of wool lessened.

Emotional dysregulation significantly reduces executive functioning and the capacity to mentalise, which can lead to further distress in the therapeutic relationship (Fonagy & Adshead, 2012). It is crucial to balance working on relational fears and the capacity to mentalise in order to fortify the therapeutic relationship. This needs to be sensitively paced and practitioners need to be mindful of not making unrealistic demands for trust or being overly reassuring as this can increase distress and anxiety and replicate abuse dynamics, leading to further disorganisation of the attachment system which can undermine the healing process and may cause harm.

Terry

Terry had been repeatedly raped by his older brother from the age of six to ten, and when he told his mother, she dismissed this as an exaggeration of normal rough and tumble play fighting rather than being a cause for concern. When Terry first entered therapy he was highly suspicious of his therapist and believed that therapists, while skilled at adopting a caring, compassionate stance, were actually 'making money out of misery'. Whenever his therapist expressed empathy in their reflections or body language, he would become inordinately enraged and scream at them that he did not want their sympathy or pity. Given the lack of empathy from either his brother or mother, and no experience of empathetic responses from his partners, he could not differentiate between empathy, sympathy, or pity. Every time empathy was shown Terry felt pitied and ashamed. It was crucial that his therapist acknowledged how hard it was for him to be in the presence of empathy and compassion as this was unbearably painful and shaming. In exploring his feeling and honouring that for Terry empathy was shaming, it was discussed how the therapist could show that they cared without triggering his shame. His therapist said that, while it would be inauthentic to suppress empathy or compassion for him, they would like to find a way of conveying this to him. Terry suggested that they moderate some of their verbal and non-verbal empathic responses and practised this to see what was more tolerable. Once Terry and his therapist agreed on what was manageable for him they explored his feelings about the SSA and how it felt for him to have it dismissed and minimised by his mother. Throughout the therapeutic work Terry found it hard to trust his therapist and their intentions and would often have to check how safe and connected he felt.

It was not until the end of the second year of therapy that Terry was able to accept the genuineness of his therapist's empathy and compassion and in turn begin to feel empathy and compassion for himself. This enabled him to become less mistrustful and suspicious, even though he remained unable to trust the therapist fully.

It was important for Terry to know that trust in others is hard to regain after such severe interpersonal trauma, and that it constantly evolves given the quality of relationships. It was important that he paced himself when trusting rather than forcing it, or being forced to by others.

Practitioners need to be aware of their own attachment histories and attachment style, as their attachment system can become hyper-activated when working with survivors or when experiencing relational difficulties in their personal life. This can equally lead to a loss of mentalising function, lack of mirroring and attunement, and impaired reflective functioning. If left unchecked, these can increase the survivor's anxiety and evoke traumatic re-enactments, or elicit practitioner defences or acting out (Sanderson, 2013).

Rather than stress the need for trust, the central focus needs to be on building a connection to counteract the disconnection and betrayal of trust inherent in SSA. It is essential that practitioners promote mutually empowering ways of engaging in relationships and embrace the restorative healing of power-in-connection (Jordan, 2000; Miller, 2015). Such connection has to be offered and not be seen as the sole responsibility of the survivor. In offering a genuinely human relationship based on mutuality, empathy, and compassion, survivors can experience relational worth and begin to connect to the self and others (Miller, 2015; Jordan, 2000). To facilitate this, TWPs need to ensure that they are authentic, visible, and fully engaged in the therapeutic process. It is helpful to regularly monitor and check with the survivor to what extent they feel connected and to be aware of signs of disconnection and withdrawal, and address these. They will need to understand that disconnection can occur for a variety of reasons, not least when the intensity of intimacy and connection becomes unbearable, necessitating the need to withdraw as a protective strategy. Survivors commonly oscillate between wanting to be connected and fearing connection, which leads to approach–avoid behaviours which need to be recognised as protective strategies (Sanderson, 2022).

Practitioners need to ensure that they remain present and attuned despite such testing behaviours and are able to track what is felt in the moment and be reflective rather than reactive. As the therapeutic relationship is integral to healing and recovery it needs to be tended with care and sensitivity, with practitioners remaining consistent and predictable, especially when survivors present with disorganised attachment style or when their lives are in a constant state of flux or chaos. Practitioners will need to guard against any potential destabilisation and ensure that they are able to tolerate uncertainty and unpredictability (Sanderson, 2013, 2022).

In order to manage any fluctuations, impasse, and ruptures in the therapeutic relationship TWPs need to demonstrate their constancy and consistency in their support of the survivor by contextualising these as protective strategies. In addition, it is essential that when there are ruptures that these are explored and the relative contribution of both parties is discussed. If some of the responsibility for the rupture lies with the practitioner it is imperative that he or she apologise. This is particularly important as survivors rarely receive apologies for the SSA or harm done to them. Receiving a genuine apology can be very healing as it reduces the tendency to blame and shame the self, or taking responsibility for other people's actions and behaviour (Sanderson, 2019). It also provides an opportunity for the practitioner to model human frailty in making errors or mistakes, and the power of apology and willingness to repair any harm done. Invariably it is the repair of the rupture that is more meaningful and healing than the actual rupture.

To ensure mutuality in the therapeutic relationship it is important for practitioners to take the initiative when a rupture occurs and to apologise for their part in this rather than wait for the rupture to metastasise or for the survivor to challenge them. Such openness and honesty is integral to feeling safe in relationships as it reduces the need to mind read. Mind reading is an indispensable skill which enables people to survive dangerous and frightening experiences as it helps them to pre-empt danger and put protective strategies in place (Sanderson, 2013, 2022). The need to mind read invariably indicates fear, confusion, or lack of safety, and necessitates the survivor exiting their frame of reference by coming out of their mind in order to enter the mind of the practitioner, and thereby losing contact with their sense of self. To avoid replicating the need to mind read, TWPs need to be explicit in their communication and encourage clarification of understanding and meaning (Sanderson, 2022).

In essence practitioners need to promote mutuality and equality in the therapeutic relationship in order to truly empower the survivor to restore relational worth and to feel safe in relationships. This needs to be accompanied with a shared understanding of the human condition and a sense of humility. Practitioners need to avoid what Maltsberger and Buie (1974) call the three narcissistic snares faced by clinicians which are 'to know all, to heal all, and to love all'. Moreover, it is when survivors feel safe in relationships that spontaneity and positive affect is restored which allows them to experience pleasure and joy in connection and intimacy rather than fear. It will also enable them to set boundaries without fear or shame so that they can flourish and grow.

To facilitate mutuality in the therapeutic relationship, practitioners need to be emotionally well regulated, somatically aware, embodied, and be able to mentalise. Through being embodied they can use their body as a tuning fork to resonate with the survivor's inner experiencing, and be aware of their own somatic reactions. It is however important not to assume anything and check any perceptions, feelings, or thoughts with the survivor.

Practitioners need to be able to track clients' somatic responses and be aware of any emotional dysregulation in order to know when to brake or accelerate exploration of distressing or shaming material (Rothschild, 2000, 2017). If the survivor becomes overwhelmed with unbearable emotions or begins to shut down or dissociate, they will not be able to mentalise or process their experiences. Rather than interpret this as resistance or non-compliance, it is crucial to see this within the context of hyper- or hypo-aroused states and the concomitant reduction in cognitive processing. This indicates the need to slow down and re-regulate before continuing further exploration. It is helpful to adopt a dyadic or co-regulation approach in which both parties demonstrate emotional self-regulation skills in order to remain present and embodied (Rothschild, 2021; Sanderson, 2022).

This is particularly the case in survivors who are unable to speak the unspeakable and cannot give voice to what happened to them or how they feel. Rather than forcing the need to use language for the benefit of the therapist who is trained in a verbally based therapeutic modality, practitioners need to consider meeting survivors at their level and working collaboratively with them to find a shared language to help make sense of what happened to them and how it affected them.

Sanna

Sanna was a child at risk from birth as she was born into a family of domestic abuse, physical violence, and substance misuse.

She was physically abused by her father while still a baby, and emotionally neglected by her mother. Sanna would often crawl into her sister's bed at night in the hope of avoiding a beating when her parents came home from the pub. While cuddled up in bed Sanna's sister would often stroke her hair to comfort her. Gradually the stroking would be extended to other parts of the body, culminating in penetration with various objects. While Sanna felt really scared, it was not as frightening as her parents and she loved her sister and would do anything for her. She couldn't tell anyone what was happening as she felt she had no voice and didn't want to get her sister into trouble, or lose her protection.

When Sanna entered therapy she could barely speak, and when she did her voice was tiny and whispery, characteristic of a small child. Her therapist often struggled to hear what she was trying to say. At other times Sanna would be mute and not able to say anything. Her therapist could see she was desperate to tell her story but couldn't find the words to express herself. The more she tried, the harder it was for her, and her shame and fear would lead her to retreat into silence. 'Talking therapy' which relies on language and words was excruciating for her. To reduce the pressure of verbal communication her therapist explored a number of ways of communicating to find what worked best for Sanna. Over a number of sessions Sanna realised that the best way for her to express herself was through drawing. At the next session Sanna started off by showing her therapist a number of drawings she had done to describe what she was feeling which her therapist then reflected back to her in words. Whenever her therapist was able to interpret this accurately, Sanna was delighted and felt safer and was able to engage a little more.

They agreed to try to use this way of communicating for the early sessions until Sanna felt more comfortable using words and language. It really felt like both client and therapist were learning a new language, Sanna learning words for feelings and sensations, and the therapist learning to decipher her emotions in drawings.

As Sanna's emotional literacy expanded she began to find her voice and express her thoughts and feelings. In activating cognitive language structures, Sanna was able to come out of the frozen pre-verbal child state and order her experiences, thoughts, and feelings so that they could be processed. By engaging with Sanna at her developmental level and reflecting words and language back to her she felt safer rather than feeling forced to find words that she didn't have.

Once her emotional literacy expanded she was able to share what happened to her and express her feelings and come out of her frozen and speechless terror.

The capacity for dual awareness along with the ability to mentalise enables practitioners to be alert and sensitive to their own as well as their client's moment-to-moment experiencing as well as modelling requisite mentalisation skills (Fonagy & Adshead, 2012). Practitioners need to facilitate mentalisation in survivors so that they are more able to understand their own mental state and the mental states of others. This is best effected through the use of reflection and the modelling of mentalisation skills that enable them to hear self and others. In addition, TWPs need to convey to the survivor that they have them in mind, both during and outside of the session, as the sense of someone having them in mind builds a bridge between sessions and reduces the sense of aloneness in the world. To ensure that the survivor is able to acquire the requisite skills to mentalise, TWPs need to make sure that they have mastered a degree of affect regulation as the capacity to mentalise is significantly weakened by intense emotions (Fonagy & Adshead, 2012).

Practitioners also need to be open-minded and be able to demonstrate flexibility and fluidity of thinking, and avoid reductionist formulations or simple solutions. They need to be able to tolerate complexity and uncertainty. This is crucial given that many survivors tend to engage in rigid, dichotomous thinking (Sanderson, 2019) and find it hard to employ more nuanced thinking. It is important not to shame survivors for their lack of flexibility in thinking as this has been a necessary strategy that has aided their survival.

A corollary to this is inflexible behaviours and boundaries. Many survivors try to obtain an illusion of control by engaging in obsessive compulsive types of behaviour that have afforded them a semblance of safety in the past, or by trying to control their environment or others. It is essential that practitioners negotiate and model healthy boundaries which are firm without being punitive, and set appropriate limits (Sanderson, 2022). These need to be consensually agreed, explicitly stated, and revised as necessary. This is particularly the case with boundaries around touch which need to be explicitly stated at the beginning of the therapeutic contract.

In order to establish an optimal therapeutic relationship despite the myriad fears around connection and intimacy, practitioners need to possess a range of relational skills that demonstrate their trustworthiness and capacity to be present. They need to be attuned, responsive, and be able to offer genuine relational warmth (Miller, 2015; Jordan, 2017). Tone of voice is a powerful way to convey attunement and needs to align with the internal self-state of the survivor. A gentle, caring tone of voice conveys to the survivor that the practitioner is empathic and responsive, whereas a loud emphatic tone of voice can induce fear, and can be misperceived as anger by the survivor. Tone of voice can also be used to regulate the survivor's level of arousal. A slow, soft, rhythmic tone of voice that is calming and soothing can reduce the level of hyper-arousal, while a slightly firmer, instructional tone of voice, emphasising the survivor's name, can bring the survivor back from a hypo-aroused state to the present.

In addition, they must be able to sustain connection and remain engaged and avoid being too abstinent as this is reminiscent of the abuse. The focus needs to be on 'being with' rather than 'doing to' and being comfortable with bearing witness to suffering, extreme terror, rage, shame, and chronic loneliness without retreating or dissociating (Sanderson, 2013, 2022). Practitioners need to be able to sustain connection and hold the unbearable pain that is too overwhelming for the survivor until they are able to do so. Rather than caretaking, TWPs need to work towards empowering the survivor to reclaim their autonomous self and restore self-agency.

In the presence of a warm, compassionate, and genuinely caring relationship survivors can learn new ways of relating to others through setting healthy boundaries, developing more effective communication skills, reflective functioning, and mentalisation. It also helps them to build mutual respect and develop relationship skills. This is a powerful antidote to their experience of relationships as a source of confusion or danger rather than a source of security, warmth, and growth. Through this, the survivor can begin to enjoy their relationships rather than fearing shame, rejection, or abandonment. This can transform their view of themselves and what it means to be connected, and thereby lead to empowerment and post-traumatic growth (Sanderson, 2022).

Support for Practitioners

Listening to and supporting survivors can be extremely harrowing and challenging, and clinicians must ensure that they are supported in their work with appropriate training, supervision, and mentoring. Research has shown that frontline professionals are impacted when working with people who experience trauma or SSA through vicarious traumatisation (VT) or compassion fatigue (CF) (Sanderson, 2013, 2022). Acknowledging and addressing this possibility, and promoting practitioner self-care strategies, minimises the risk of burnout or secondary traumatic stress (STS).

Working with survivors of SSA raises a number of challenges such as assessment and safeguarding issues, as well as a fear of re-traumatisation. In addition, some practitioners find it hard to believe some of the abuse experiences and find it difficult to bear witness to the survivor's lived experience. A further challenge is becoming aroused when listening to the survivor's experiences. Practitioners need to be mindful that such arousal is not necessarily sexual, but may represent fear and alarm which has been eroticised, which mirrors the survivor's experience (Sanderson, 2019). It is crucial that practitioners are able to take this to supervision, preferably with a trauma trained supervisor, to get the requisite support.

To protect themselves from the negative impact of caring for others it is helpful for practitioners to develop an understanding and increased awareness of their own symptoms of burnout, CF, VT, and STS. This will enable them to check-in regularly with their emotional and psychological well-being and to track levels of emotional and physical depletion in order to put strategies in place to manage these and prevent further decompensation. Saakvitne and Pearlman (1996) suggest that practitioners develop a personalised warning system which enables them to recognise and identify CF/STS symptoms on a scale of 1 to 10 (with 10 being the worst they have ever felt about their work, empathy, and compassion, and 1 the best). To facilitate this, practitioners can adopt a traffic light system to identify the top three physical, emotional, and behavioural warning signs that indicate disruptions to their well-being, and when to implement effective strategies before symptoms worsen (Saakvitne & Pearlman, 1996).

To minimise VT it is crucial to take regular physical as well as mental breaks, to exercise regularly to keep up energy levels, and to remain embodied. Practitioners need to counterbalance trauma work with activities that restore any shattered beliefs they may have about the world by engaging in activities that help them to regain faith in human nature, and restore vitality, enthusiasm, and energy. This will also enable them to remain connected to self and others so that they are more able to bear witness to and fully support survivors of SSA in their journey to recovery and healing.

Regular monitoring of personal and professional functioning ensures that practitioners are robust and resilient enough to manage the demands and challenges of working with clients without feeling diminished or depleted. This needs to be accompanied by a range of strategies that will recalibrate their physical, emotional, and psychological well-being. To effect this, practitioners are encouraged to consider a range of self-care strategies and how these can be implemented both during sessions, post session, and in their personal life. Skovholt and Trotter-Mathison (2016) emphasise the need to focus on being a 'good enough counsellor' who is well bounded and able to manage both client and practitioner expectations. In addition, practitioners are encouraged to establish a consistent and reliable support network that includes regular supervision, peer supervision, as well as positive and enriching interactions with colleagues and co-workers (Sanderson, 2013).

It is essential that practitioners implement work-related as well as personal self-care strategies in order to maintain a balance between professional identity and personal values throughout the caring process. In order to manage the demand of the work they need to ensure that the work remains meaningful and that they are able to set realistic goals (Sanderson, 2013, 2022). In addition, they need to be able to create a comfortable and safe work environment and have a sense of self-efficacy with regard to the number of clients in their caseload, the number of sessions per day, and length of break between each client. For example, it can be helpful to schedule the most complex or demanding clients in a block either at the beginning or at the end of the week, or at a time of day when the practitioner is most alert, energised, and focused (Skovholt & Trotter-Mathison, 2016).

Practitioners will also need to set appropriate boundaries for their clients and themselves, through setting limits, being able to say no without feeling guilty, working reasonable hours, taking regular breaks, and counterbalancing client work with other professional activities such as training, teaching, writing, research, or promoting mental health through some form of activism. In addition, they need to ensure regular supervision and continuous professional development training to extend their knowledge and enhance confidence (Sanderson, 2013).

There are a range of self-care skills that practitioners can employ both during and immediately after the session which can ensure that they stay grounded and present. During the session it is helpful to have an anchor in the room for the practitioner to ground themselves mentally as well as physically, in order to remain embodied. In addition, practitioners need to be aware of the somatic impact in their body through body scans to check for any tension, or somatic reactions, and to monitor signs of somatic countertransference (Sanderson, 2013). In incorporating regular self-care strategies, practitioners will be able to remain embodied and present when working with survivors and be able to facilitate the survivor's healing and post-traumatic growth.

The next chapter will explore the range of protective factors that mitigate the risk of being subjected to SSA, as well as reducing the risk of children committing HSB. It will also examine the importance of working with families to improve understanding of HSB, how to set clear boundaries, ensure adequate supervision of children, and how to talk about sex with children and adolescents in an age appropriate way.

Further Reading

Cozolino, L. (2021). *The development of a therapist: Healing others – healing self* (Kindle edn). W.W. Norton.
Herman, J.L. (2001). *Trauma and recovery* (2nd edn). Basic Books.
Jordan, J.V. (2017). *Relational-cultural therapy* (2nd edn). American Psychological Association.

Jordan, J.V. (2017). Relational-cultural theory: The power of connection to transform our lives. *The Journal of Humanistic Counselling*, 56, 3.

Miller, J.B. (2015). *The healing connection: How women form relationships in therapy and in life*. Beacon Press.

One in Four. (2015). *Survivors' voices*. One in Four.

One in Four. (2019). *Numbing the pain*. One in Four.

Rothschild, B. (2017). *The body remembers. Volume 2: Revolutionizing trauma treatment*. W.W. Norton.

Sanderson, C. (2013). *Counselling skills for working with trauma*. Jessica Kingsley Publishers.

Sanderson, C. (2015). *Counselling skills for working with shame*. Jessica Kingsley Publishers.

Sanderson, C. (2015). *Responding to survivors of child sexual abuse: A pocket guide for professionals, partners, families and friends*. One in Four.

Sanderson, C. (2022). *The warrior within: A One in Four handbook to aid recovery for survivors of childhood sexual abuse and violence* (4th edn). One in Four.

Smith, N., Dogaru, C., & Ellis, F. (2015). *Hear me. Believe me. Respect me. A survey of adult survivors of child sexual abuse and their experience of support services*. University Campus Suffolk.

Van der Kolk, B. (2015). *The body keeps the score: Mind, brain and body in the transformation of trauma*. Penguin Books.

Zaleski, K.L., Johnson, D.K., & Klein, J.T. (2016). Grounding Judith Herman's trauma theory within interpersonal neuroscience and evidence-based practice modalities for trauma treatment. *Smith College Studies in Social Work*, 86(4), 377–393.

CHAPTER 11

The Prevention of Sibling Sexual Abuse

Preventing and minimising the risk of SSA requires the raising of public and professional awareness. This chapter will explore the range of factors that can protect children from SSA and minimise the risk of children committing HSB. It will look at the importance of working with families to improve understanding of SSA and HSB, how to set clear boundaries, ensure adequate supervision of children, and how to talk to children and adolescents about sex in an age appropriate way. It is hoped that with increased awareness of SSA among professionals including social workers, child protection workers, youth workers, the police, and teachers, as well as mental health practitioners and therapists, that children in families will be more adequately protected.

The prevention of SSA is most effectively addressed from an early age at an individual level through the family and the community, schools, and society (Letourneau et al., 2017). This needs to be conducted using a holistic, child-focused, and strengths-based approach that involves all those affected by SSA, including family work. This is best achieved through integrated and regulated agency responses (Hackett, 2004, 2014; Smith et al., 2013) which focuses on meeting the needs of all those involved and affected by SSA, including parents, carers, teachers, children's services, and youth justice intervention, as well as access to specialist care (Hackett et al., 2014).

Preventative Approaches

Research and awareness of SSA is nominal compared to intergenerational child sexual abuse which has significant consequences with regard to identification and assessment of SSA, appropriate responses and intervention, as well as prevention. The lack of knowledge of what constitutes inter-sibling sexual abuse means parents, teachers, health professionals, and the community are not clear on how to respond or how to seek help or support. This leads to under-reporting and the minimisation of SSA as a less harmful form of abuse which does not warrant serious public health attention. There needs to be a significant social and policy shift in order to provide appropriate support and service provision.

Policy Changes

The lack of definition and clear national guidelines or protocols serves to minimise SSA and renders it a hidden form of abuse which cannot be legitimised. It is imperative that SSA is seen as a form of interpersonal violence between siblings which is predicated on the misuse of power and control, sense of entitlement, and sexual privilege, which reflects patriarchal ideologies and the objectification of children (Caffaro, 2017, 2020). The provision of national guidelines will aid reporting and disclosure and effective support for siblings who have been harmed and those who have harmed, as well as parents and families.

Given the role of trauma in families who are at risk of SSA, it is prudent to implement routine screening for ACEs, trauma, HSB, as well as SSA. Good practice guidelines that emphasise attachment and use a relational and trauma-informed approach will help when supporting families and the sibling dyad to find the most optimal interventions, and the most effective therapeutic outcomes. In addition, policy change needs to incorporate specialist training programmes for professionals working with children or adult survivors to understand the complexity of SSA, and gain a deeper understanding of the harmful impact and long-term effects. In acknowledging the seriousness of SSA practitioners will need to have access to regular case supervision and/or mentoring to manage the impact of working with SSA (McCartan et al., 2021).

Public Health Education Campaign

Policy changes can also be supported by psychoeducation through public health education to inform parents, families, teachers, professionals, children, and adult survivors about the nature of SSA and promote change in social attitudes. This needs to include awareness that not all sibling relationships are benign and nurturing and that some are harmful, especially when there is an abuse of power and control, or coercive non-consensual sexual activity (see Box 11.1). In addition, there needs to be psychoeducation on what is considered developmentally typical sexual curiosity and sexual play and what constitutes developmentally atypical sexual behaviour so the two can be distinguished. Guidance should also include how early exposure to pornography can lead to the re-enactment of sexual behaviour between siblings or peers, and how parents can monitor this and approach talking about it with their children. In addition, parents need to be aware of the vulnerability of neurodivergent children to being sexually harmed, or committing HSB and SSA, and how to mitigate this.

Any public health campaign needs to be supported with clear guidelines regarding reporting the SSA to the relevant agencies and signposting to sources of help for the sibling dyad as well as other siblings and the family. Parents and families need to be assured that they will be listened to and heard without being blamed for the SSA, and that they will be supported throughout. Siblings who have been harmed as well as siblings who have harmed need to know that they will be supported, and those with dual status will be responded to in an empathic and compassionate way. Adult survivors also need to be signposted to specialist services where they can give voice and will be heard without being dismissed or having the SSA minimised or normalised.

Box 11.1 Summary of public education messages

- Raise awareness of HSB, TA-HSB, and SSA and its impact and how this differs from CSA
- Clear definition of what constitutes SSA
- Awareness that SSA is estimated to be three times more common than intergenerational CSA
- Differences between developmentally typical and atypical sexual behaviour
- Signs of SSA
- Vulnerability to SSA in children who are neurodivergent or have learning difficulties
- Role of trauma and ACEs that increase risk of SSA
- Recognise that some children who commit SSA may have 'dual status' in having been sexually abused themselves

- Family factors that elevate the risk of committing SSA
- Impact of early exposure to pornography and link to SSA
- Reporting guidance
- Sources of support for the sibling who is being harmed and sibling who has harmed and families
- Support services for adult survivors

Media
Public health campaigns can be amplified by media coverage through the ethical reporting of SSA through news stories, discussion on TV or radio programmes or talk shows, documentaries, podcasts, or streaming platforms. In addition, films and television dramas can fulfil an important function by developing storylines which include HSB and SSA, especially in TV series or soap dramas. The effectiveness of psychoeducation through TV drama has been demonstrated in the coverage of storylines involving domestic abuse, sexual violence and rape, and child sexual abuse.

Community-Based Programmes
Community-based programmes that emphasise healthy family relationships could also address the nature of sibling relationships as well as the potential of physical or sexual abuse by siblings. Community workers can monitor behaviour of siblings and remain vigilant about behaviour that is cause for concern. In offering sibling-focused prevention practices they can enhance sibling relationships by promoting pro-social sibling interactions through shared constructive activities, developing perspective-taking skills, and reducing relational aggression, which in turn can improve other family relationships (Caffaro, 2017).

School Education Programmes
School-based programmes are ideally placed to raise awareness of the nature of healthy relationships, the importance of mutual respect, and setting appropriate boundaries. They also provide opportunities to talk about unhealthy attitudes and behaviours, feelings of safety and fear, or challenges children and young people encounter in their relationships with peers and family members, including siblings. In the safe environment of school they can explore issues around consent and the digitisation of sexual behaviours, including pornography. In offering

their support, teachers can help children and young people to increase their knowledge about appropriate and inappropriate sexual behaviour, gain confidence to talk about their experiences, and give voice to any concerns they may have around sexuality and sexual behaviours.

Age appropriate sexual abuse prevention programmes that are taught across the curriculum from primary school level through to secondary and tertiary level are thought to be more effective than short-term programmes in mitigating inappropriate sexual behaviour (Hackett et al., 2019), especially when they involve young people in their development and delivery (Caffaro, 2017). This can be combined with sex education, and discussions about consent, sexual objectification, safe sex, and the impact of exposure to pornography and the use of cyber-sex, as well as technology-assisted harmful sexual behaviour, and issues of privilege, power, and entitlement.

Schools could further extend some of these programmes to outreach projects and involve parents by offering psychoeducation sessions, to increase their awareness of the landscape of sexuality and sexual behaviours among young people, including the nature of SSA, how to set boundaries and ensure adequate supervision, as well as safeguarding policies, reporting guidelines, and pastoral support. While there is insufficient research data on the effectiveness of school programmes with regard to SSA, they do offer the opportunity to counter attitudes that legitimise harmful sexual behaviours.

Professionals

All professionals who come into contact with children and families, including social workers, child protection workers, child development specialists, mental health care professionals, therapists, teachers, police, and youth offending teams, will benefit from increased awareness of SSA. It is critical that they are apprised of the complexity of SSA and the interplay of trauma, individual and familial risk factors, dysfunctional family dynamics, and socio-cultural factors, and how these relate to negative mental and physical health outcomes. They also need to have an understanding of the nature of sibling relationships and not assume that they are always benign and nurturing. Such training will also ensure that all professionals working in partnership or within a multi-agency framework are equally knowledgeable and thereby reduce confusion or conflict among workers to facilitate more accurate assessments and interventions.

Specialist training has to be supported with evidence-based guidelines to fully understand the impact and seriousness of HSB and SSA (Hackett et al., 2014; Allardyce & Yates, 2013 Yates, 2018; Yates & Allardyce, 2022) to ensure that these are not normalised or minimised. Professionals also need to be able to distinguish between benign, playful, sexual curiosity, and SSA (Turner et al., 2010). It will also help to recognise that even if a child does not view the SSA as abusive, or there are no overt signs of harm, that this does not mean that harm is not being committed, and if there is no intervention, that the SSA can escalate. Equipped with such knowledge they can extend the appropriate support when SSA is disclosed and mitigate the risk of further re-traumatisation or post-disclosure trauma.

Parents and Families
Parents and carers can also play an essential role in the prevention of SSA, providing they are equipped with knowledge and information that helps them to understand and identify SSA, and know how best to support their children, and how to access emotional and psychological support (Bovarnick & Scott, 2016).

Professionals can share their specialist knowledge to educate parents to have a greater understanding of the nature of SSA and how to manage disclosure and how to support both siblings. They can also become role models for pro-social behaviour and help parents to develop more positive parent-to-child and sibling-to-sibling relationships, set appropriate boundaries, and promote more healthy family relationships. This can include positive ways to challenge aggressive or abusive behaviour, how to mediate sibling conflicts and ensure that they provide adequate supervision of siblings and their behaviour (Hackett, 2001; Smith et al., 2014). It is also helpful to discuss the negative impact of physical punishment and its relation to later aggression or violence, and promote alternative forms of moderating children's behaviours.

Parents can also learn ways in which they can develop non-intrusive supervision and how to monitor what children watch on TV and their devices. Rather than let children passively watch films, TV programmes, or social media posts, it is helpful to talk to them about their thoughts and feelings in response to what they have watched. This enables them to process the material and is a fruitful way of exploring associated issues around sexuality and sexual behaviour.

How to Talk about Sex in an Age Appropriate Way

One way of equipping parents to prevent SSA is to help them find ways to have an open channel of communication with their children from early childhood about bodies, boundaries and personal space, appropriate and inappropriate touching, and to know and express when they feel safe or unsafe. This can lead into being able to talk about sex in an age appropriate way (see Table 11.1).

To do this they need to be aware of changing attitudes towards gender, sexuality, and sexual practices including gender fluidity, sexual identity, range of sexual preferences and the impact of social media, posting of sexual images, cyber-sex, and early exposure to pornography. Parents can be a reliable source of information around sex and sexuality providing they themselves are knowledgeable and they are not too inhibited to talk about sex with their children (Sanderson, 2004).

When talking about sex it is crucial that parents let their children know they can talk about anything related to their body, including feeling confused or fearful, without being shamed, or being made to feel guilty or dirty, and without fear of punishment. It helps the child to know that it is important to be aware of their body and bodily signals, which helps them to know whether they feel safe or not, and this develops emotional, somatic, and sexual literacy in expressing what they think and feel. In addition, they need to know that they can say 'No' when touch feels confusing or uncomfortable, or when they feel their personal space is being invaded (Sanderson, 2004).

To make talking about sex easier, parents can use cues in their psychosocial world such as someone known to the child being pregnant, or something they have seen on TV or in a film or music video, on social media, or a celebrity news story. Using these as prompts they can encourage the child to ask questions and respond to these in a calm and collected way, as they would any other question about the child's world. Such conversations do not need to be lengthy information feeds; they are more effective if they are in bite-size chunks and confined to answering specific questions. It is not necessary to fit everything into one conversation, and remember that little but often is more likely to satisfy the child's curiosity, and it can always be reinforced at a later time if necessary. It is important to use age appropriate language that the child can comprehend and make sense of, and be child-led with regard to any questions they have.

Table 11.1 Summary of how to talk to children about sex

0–24 months	2–4-year-olds	5–8-year-olds	9–12-year-olds	Teenagers
Name body parts	Touching rules	Expand on body parts and internal reproductive system	Talk about puberty – hormonal and bodily changes	Consolidate what has been learnt
Difference between boys and girls	Privacy	How bodies are different	Expand on range of sexual behaviours	How to navigate dating
Functions of the body	Boundaries	Look after their body	Attraction and sexual fantasy	Use of pornography
Label feelings	Body ownership	Rehearse saying 'no'	Discuss dating and healthy relationships	Online sex – risk of sextortion
Touch – good and bad	Set limits around sexual play	Puberty	Sexual values	Posting sexual images
Talk about not keeping secrets	Talk about reproduction	Sexual intercourse as part of sexual reproduction	Consent	Filming sexual activities
Set boundaries	Don't keep secrets around the body	Kissing, hugging, touching	Discuss safe sex	Revenge porn
	Talk about anything that is confusing	Sexual boundaries	Pornography	Consent
	Rehearse safety behaviour scenarios	Masturbation	How to be cyber-smart	Sexual preferences
	Read books	Sexual images	Gender dysmorphia – transgender	Safe sex
		Range of gender identities and sexual orientations	How to manage peer pressure	Dangers of intoxication
				Intimacy and relationships

Some parents will find it difficult to talk about sex with their children and may benefit from practising with their partner or a trusted friend (Sanderson, 2004). In addition, professionals could consider running small group workshops for parents where they can practise talking about sex and how to respond to their children. Practising such conversations first can make it easier for parents to manage any discomfort or unease, which will help children to feel less uncomfortable about expressing themselves, and avoid them shutting down.

Open communication of feelings and problems and listening to the child will set a precedent which can make it easier for them to seek advice in the future as they grow older. It will also equip them with appropriate knowledge about how to develop healthy relationships built on mutual trust and respect, the rights and responsibilities of partners in romantic relationships, and how to act appropriately.

It is crucial to remember that children have different questions and concerns about sex at different ages, and as they develop and mature. The questions that children ask signpost parents to what they already know and the things they wish to talk about. It is important to listen attentively even if the parent doesn't agree with the child's opinion, and be honest about how they feel. Parents need to monitor their own inhibitions and try to avoid showing any embarrassment.

Talking about good and bad touch is important, along with an acknowledgement that touch in certain parts of the body feels nice, and can sometimes be confusing. Parents need to teach their children that their body belongs to them and that they have a right to express themselves if they don't like something such as being pinched, squeezed, hugged, or kissed. In allowing them to express how they feel and to say 'no' parents are equipping them with the necessary skills to protect themselves. Being able to say 'no' and strategies of how to manage situations that are confusing or uncomfortable can be rehearsed with the parent to help the child when they feel they are in danger (Sanderson, 2004).

How to Talk to Children Age 0–24 Months

Although children at this stage are largely pre-verbal, they are still able to learn about their bodies through parents talking to them. The goal when talking to children this young is to help them feel comfortable with their whole body without shame. Children are naturally curious about their bodies, and those of others, and want to explore their bodies. Parents can help them to name body parts, preferably using correct anatomical terms such as penis, vagina, or vulva, and talk about bodily functions such as urinating or excreting, and anatomical differences between boys and girls. To help develop somatic and emotional literacy parents need to label sensations and feelings and acknowledge what feels nice, what feels uncomfortable, or what feels confusing. It is important to let children know that they can touch all parts of their body so that they can experience what feels good and what feels bad. This can segue into talking about boundaries in an age appropriate way, such as discussing hugging, kissing, nudity, and touching intimate parts of the body, and that if they feel confused or uncomfortable with others touching them, they are allowed to say that they don't like that.

How to Talk to Children Age 2-4
As children become more verbal they will ask more questions about their bodies and are more able to express what they are feeling. Parents can now expand on the previous developmental stage by talking more about boundaries and privacy to encourage the child's sense of ownership over their bodies, and to make it clear they do not need to keep any secrets around their body. This includes boundaries around touch and that while the touching of their genitals is perfectly normal, it is best not to do so in public. The respect for privacy is not only for the child but the privacy of others, and they must not touch or hug others if the other person feels uncomfortable. The emphasis is on being able to say they don't like it if someone touches, hugs, or kisses them in a way that is confusing, and equally to respect others if they say no to being touched. This can be combined with talking about what to do if someone touches them in a way that is confusing, or makes them do something they don't want to do, which can be practised and rehearsed. It is also important to let them know that no-one should ask them to keep secrets about their body or sexual play and that they can tell a parent if they are told to do this (Sanderson, 2004).

As this is the stage where children engage in developmentally normal sexual exploration with other children, it is nevertheless important to set appropriate boundaries and ensure that they engage in a broad range of play activities, not just sexual play (Sanderson, 2004). At this age children will also become curious about where babies come from. Parents need to answer their questions and convey basic concepts such as babies are made by combining an egg with sperm, and that the baby grows inside a mummy's tummy, and comes out through the vagina. It is important to stress that making babies is something that adults do, not something that children do, no matter what anyone tells them. To make it easier for parents to talk about bodies and reproduction with children there are a number of excellent age appropriate books that can be read together, for example:

- *Pantosaurus and the Power of PANTS!* (Gerlings & Galloway, 2021)
- *It's My Body: A Book about Body Privacy for Young Children* (Spilsbury, 2020)
- *My Underpants Rule* (Power & Power, 2014)
- *Hello, World! My Body* (McDonald, 2018)
- *Whisper* (Waddell & Waddell, 2016)
- *Share Some Secrets* (Gabbitas, 2014)

How to Talk to Children Age 5–8
As children get older they will want to expand their knowledge about their bodies and reproductive functions. This is in part due to greater cognitive understanding but also through an ever expanding psychosocial world and exposure to social media, TV, news stories, films, books, and music. This is a time when parents can build on the previous stage by expanding on the function of different body parts and the internal reproductive system. Discussions about sexual intercourse as part of sexual reproduction is crucial, and it should be conveyed that this is a natural and normal part of healthy adult relationships, and that adults can choose whether to have a child. It is also important to convey that sexual intercourse is only one of many ways to show how adults care for each other, not the only way. It is essential to emphasise the importance of healthy relationships and intimacy, and not just sexual activities. Children at this stage will discover that masturbation feels good, and they need to be reminded that this is healthy and normal.

 Children at this age also become more aware of differences in bodies with regard to shape, size, colour, and gender, as well as gender identity and sexual orientation. It is crucial that parents are able to talk openly about this, even if they don't fully understand gender and sexual diversity, or approve of it. They need to emphasise that there are many different ways to express love and with different people irrespective of gender.

 Research shows that some children as young as eight will be exposed to sexual images by peers. Parents will need to discuss that while some adults do look at naked images, or watch sexual activity on the internet, this is not designed for children, and help their child with strategies of what to do if they feel pressurised to look at sexual images, or are coerced to post such images themselves, or to film younger siblings.

How to Talk to Children Age 9–12
Most children enter puberty during this stage and the focus will be on hormonal and body changes. Parents can prepare children for puberty by talking to their children about how their bodies will change as they develop secondary sex characteristics, and how hormonal changes can affect their mood and sense of well-being. Many children have anxieties during puberty which can be exacerbated if they do not know what is happening to them, or if they feel that they are early or late developers compared to their peers.

Parents will need to be aware of when their children enter puberty and will need to talk to female children about menstruation and becoming sexually reproductive and how to manage this, as well as bodily changes and understanding these. Male children will experience ejaculation when they masturbate, and nocturnal emissions which they often feel embarrassed about. It is important to talk about these and help them recognise that this is normal, as are changes in their body and voice. Parents also need to discuss that as they become sexually mature they need to ensure that they look after themselves with regard to personal hygiene and safe sex if they should become sexually active. In addition, parents need to reassure them that fluctuating moods are due to hormonal changes. Some children will experience gender dysphoria, and parents need to be understanding and supportive of this.

As children enter puberty they will have more questions about sexual behaviours, sexual intercourse, and associated concerns such as around safe sex, contraception, and sexually transmitted infections. Parents need to respond to these concerns and seize the opportunity to talk about crushes and sexual attraction, dating, the role of consent, sexual values and beliefs, the range of sexual acts, and what feels safe for them. Children who have been exposed to pornography may believe that they have to copy the same sexual acts that they have viewed, and it is important for parents to remind them that the sexual acts in pornography are exaggerated and not representative of sexual behaviour within a loving healthy relationship. It is also important to guide them how to be cyber-smart and to avoid being sexually exploited online, or being enticed into sexual activities against their will.

How to Talk to Teenagers

This is the time for consolidating everything that has been discussed and learnt, and to explore more complex and nuanced aspects of dating and sexual behaviour. Parents will need to be available to talk about dating and to offer support in the case of unrequited attraction, rejection, or break-up. It is important to remind teenagers about consent and that both parties have a responsibility to not have sex with someone who is unable to consent, due to intoxication or because they are comatose, and that they can say no if they wish to. To facilitate this conversation it can be helpful to watch the Tea and Consent video (Blue Seat Studios, 2015).

Further discussion and guidance around the posting of sexual images, filming sexual encounters, or engaging in online sex is also prudent given the risk of sextortion. Young people need to be aware of being unknowingly filmed while engaging in online sex and how this can be used to extort money from them. The danger of filming any sexual activity is that this can be distributed online and via social media to shame the individual as in revenge porn, or to exploit them financially. It is also important to continue to talk about pornography and how it is a form of entertainment which exaggerates sexual behaviour and does not represent the intimacy, respect, or care and affection intrinsic in healthy romantic relationships.

Teenagers will also be exploring their sexual identity and sexual preferences and may need to talk about sexual fluidity, LGBTQIA+ issues, and sexual practices and acts, and parents need to be available to talk about this. Alongside this they need to reiterate the importance of safe sex, contraception, and what to do if they or their partner get pregnant. Parents also need to talk with their teenager about how to be safe and the dangers of intoxication through drugs or alcohol, and the risk of drinks being spiked, and sexual assault. As the teenager reaches adulthood the focus needs to be on safety in sexual situations or relationships, and equipping them with the knowledge of what to do if they are in danger, how to resist being pressurised into sex, and what to do if they are sexually assaulted or raped.

Challenges in Talking about Sex

Talking to children about sex can be challenging due to parents' own inhibitions, and yet it helps to keep children safe, facilitates appropriate sexual behaviour, and reduces the risk of further re-victimisation. It is important that parents are aware of their own attitudes and beliefs about sexuality and sexual orientation. To talk openly parents will need to overcome their own inhibitions and any feelings of embarrassment or shame. The more comfortable they feel talking about sex the easier it is for the child to talk to the parent. Equipping the child with accurate knowledge means that they are less vulnerable to being groomed by a sibling, peer, or adult. It will also make it easier for them to disclose any inappropriate sexual advances or activities that are uncomfortable or confusing.

Ideally in families where there are two parents or carers, it helps if both parents are able to talk to the children, and they agree on what is discussed. In single parent families, the parent may find it helpful to practise with a trusted friend or a family case worker. If a child does disclose sexual abuse it is important that parents validate the child's experience and seek out professional help and support.

Professionals may also find it challenging to talk about sex, or bear witness to graphic sexual descriptions of sexual abuse, due to their own inhibitions and beliefs around children's sexuality. They need to be aware of sexual development in children and what is typical and atypical sexual behaviour, and what constitutes HSB and SSA. This is crucial so that they do not minimise or catastrophise SSA. Overall, open communication with children and young people when talking about sexuality and listening to them, without judgement or shame, can help children to give voice to their thoughts, feelings, and experiences. This enables them to make sense of their psychosocial world and what happens to them in it, increases their sense of safety, and reduces risk of further re-victimisation.

Building on this chapter, the next chapter will identify areas for future research and how to improve professional practice through establishing a clear definition of SSA, and developing national guidelines for assessment and treatment intervention. This will increase awareness of SSA among professionals such as social care workers, child protection workers, youth workers, the police, and teachers, as well as mental health professionals, psychologists, and therapists. This in combination with specialist training will ensure that professionals are appropriately resourced to support children, families, and adult survivors of SSA.

Further Reading

Allardyce, S., & Yates, P. (2018). *Working with children and young people who have displayed harmful sexual behaviour*. Dunedin.

Caffaro, J. (2020). Sibling abuse of other children. In R. Geffner, V. Vieth, V. Vaughan-Eden, A. Rosenbaum, L. Hamberger, & J. White (eds), *Handbook of Interpersonal Violence across the Lifespan*. Springer.

Caffaro, J.V., & Conn-Caffaro, A. (1998). *Sibling abuse trauma: Assessment and intervention strategies for children, families and adults*. Routledge.

Hackett, S., Balfe, M., Masson, H., & Phillips, J. (2014). Family responses to young people who have sexually abused: Anger, ambivalence and acceptance. *Children & Society*, *28*(2), 128–139.

McCartan, K., Anning, A., & Qureshi, E. (2021). *The impact of sibling sexual abuse on adults who were harmed as children*. UWE, Bristol Research Report.

Yates, P. (2017). Sibling sexual abuse: Why don't we talk about it? *Journal of Clinical Nursing*, *26*(15-16), 2482–2494.

Yates, P., & Allardyce, S. (2021). *Sibling sexual abuse: Knowledge and practice*. Centre of Expertise on Child Sexual Abuse.

Yates, P., & Allardyce, S. (2022). Abuse at the heart of the family: The challenges and complexities of sibling sexual abuse. In K. Uzieblo, W.J. Smid, & K. McCartan (eds), *Challenges in the Management of People Convicted of a Sexual Offence*. Palgrave Macmillan.

Yates, P., & Allardyce, S. (2022). Young people who sexually harm others. In R. Clawson, R. Fryson, & L. Warwick (eds), *The Child Protection Handbook* (4th edn). Elsevier.

CHAPTER 12

Future Research and Professional Practice

To reduce and prevent SSA requires more research with regard to formulating a definition, developing robust risk assessment protocols, and clear reporting guidelines. This chapter will identify future areas for research including more clinical research with regard to interventions for all concerned and how individuals and families can best be supported, whether through individual therapy, family systems therapy, or group work. More empirical research is also needed to understand the nature of SSA, the range of motivations, and the relative contribution of a history of sexual abuse, trauma, individual factors, family dynamics, and socio-cultural factors.

With the increase of the digitisation of sex and ease of access to pornography, it is imperative that research investigates the link between early exposure to pornography and SSA. It is likely that in watching pornography some children will seek to copy or imitate what they have seen and entice younger children or siblings to re-enact this. Such research also needs to take into consideration the impact of peer pressure to watch pornography, or film and post sexual images of themselves, or younger siblings performing sexual acts.

As SSA can have lifelong consequences, future research also needs to encompass the impact of SSA, common signs and symptoms, and the long-term effects in adulthood. Qualitative research such as McCartan et al. (2021) will provide the lived experience of survivors and contribute to improving reporting procedures, responses to disclosure, and access to service provision.

The experience of dual status children also warrants further research so that more protective and preventive strategies can be put in place, and to ensure they have access to specialist therapeutic support as well as being held accountable for the harm they have caused. This includes appropriate support during adulthood so that they are more able to manage the dissonance between having committed SSA as a child and their sense of self as an adult, especially as they become parents themselves and face safeguarding procedures.

Other fruitful areas for research include the relative contribution of family dynamics that elevate the risk of SSA, including parent's history of sexual abuse in childhood, either intergenerationally or by a sibling, or having committed SSA themselves (Yates & Allardyce, 2021).

Future research will improve awareness and understanding of SSA across a number of sectors, including among the public, to clarify what structures need to be put in place to support all those who have been impacted by it, including professionals, as well as shaping effective prevention and intervention strategies.

Professional Practice

Good practice in cases of SSA needs to focus on safety planning and access to support from people who can help siblings stay safe. These can include family members, carers, and professionals such as child protection and family case workers, community-based youth workers, teachers, and mental health specialists (Courtois & Ford, 2012). There is considerable agreement that a multi-agency approach is most effective, especially if supported by a family systems approach which combines developmental, attachment, and relational perspectives (McCartan et al., 2021; Yates & Allardyce, 2022), and is tailored to each family's particular needs. Given the role of trauma in SSA, this is best delivered within a trauma-informed practice approach, that contains the principles of the Power Threat Meaning Framework in focusing on what happened to the sibling who is being harmed and sibling who has harmed, rather than on what is wrong with them, and how they had to adapt to survive and make meaning of their experiences (Johnstone & Boyle, 2018; Boyle & Johnstone, 2020; Sanderson, 2022).

Family Interventions

Despite the agreed value of family work, once a disclosure of SSA is made, professionals will face numerous challenges and encounter difficult decisions with respect to risk assessment, safety of sibling living or contact arrangements, and any potential conflicts among family members. Parental feelings can lead to divided loyalties and negative reactions towards the sibling who is being harmed and the sibling who has harmed, as well as blame directed towards their partner. It is important to acknowledge the complexity of familial reactions and ensure that all those involved are appropriately supported. A multi-agency approach which provides psychoeducation on SSA and its impact on each individual and the rest of the family has been shown to be beneficial, especially if it includes discussion of boundaries around the body, physical touch, and the rights and responsibilities of each sibling (McCartan et al., 2021). While multi-agency work is beneficial it is not always easy as there may be a range of views and reactions to SSA and how it is managed which can cause conflict and impede how families are supported. To mitigate the complex challenges inherent in multi-agency and multi-disciplinary collaboration and the coordination of services requires ongoing specialised training and skills to ensure all professionals are equally resourced.

Family systems therapy has been shown to have generally positive effects as long as it is safe and therapeutic alliances with each family member have been established. It is also helpful to explore family dynamics during family group therapy sessions, and as long as it is safe it can, in some cases, preserve the family unit. However, it is crucial to provide other support structures around the sibling who is being harmed including trauma-informed therapeutic practice (McCartan et al., 2021).

If the risk of continued harm is high, or when the level of emotional distress is too overwhelming for the sibling who is being harmed, professionals need to decide whether the siblings can remain under the same roof. They will need to assess the likelihood of further harm, or the escalation of the abuse, to what extent the family physical environment is safe with regard to number of bedrooms, bathroom faculties, power imbalances wherein older siblings have responsibilities to look after younger siblings, attitudes toward sexuality and nudity, and whether the parents have adequate protective capacities and are able to implement these (Yates & Allardyce, 2021). In addition, appropriate arrangements need to be made for sibling contact, and for supervised contact.

In supporting families, professionals need to be sensitive to socio-cultural factors such as race, religion, cultural expectations, and socio-economic status in how they shape family identities and responses to family discord. This needs to be balanced with acknowledgement of the strengths and resources different cultures can provide (Caffaro, 2020).

Interventions for Siblings Who Have Committed Sibling Sexual Abuse

To assess children who engage in HSB professionals use the Assessment Intervention Moving On (AIM36) assessment, which recommends intensive specialist treatment along with community-based long-term support, brief focused educative programmes, and parental support when the level of concern is low (Hackett et al., 2014). This is often supported by the Good Lives Model, which is a strengths-based model which emphasises the need to resource children and young people from 6 to 18 to develop and implement life changes through psychoeducation around boundaries and personal space, devising safety plans, life story work, cost and benefit analyses of HSB, and goal setting and implementation (Ward, 2002).

Research on the effectiveness of interventions is still inconclusive, although there is some evidence that cognitive behavioural and resilience models, along with multi-systemic interventions, can benefit some children and young people who engage in HSB (Masson and Hackett, 2003; Ward et al., 2007) and decrease the risk of re-offending (Campbell, 2016). These could be adapted to working with siblings who commit SSA as long as they are non-judgemental and non-shaming by focusing on 'what has happened to the child' rather than 'what is wrong with the child' (Johnstone & Boyle, 2018).

It is also not clear to what extent structured, holistic, and family-oriented approaches benefit younger children who display HSB, especially if they have a history of sexual abuse. While developmentally appropriate behavioural or cognitive behavioural approaches can be of benefit, they need to be integrated within trauma-informed and multi-systemic practice which involves both the child and the family (Saunders et al., 2003) and promotes healthy and enduring relationships (Hackett et al., 2013).

Interventions for siblings who have committed SSA, especially those who have dual status, need to include support from professionals who are empathic, compassionate, and non-judgemental, and who can offer consistent continuity of care to enable them to develop stable and enduring relationships to restore relational worth and acquire the necessary skills to have healthy relationships (Hackett et al., 2014). In addition, research on HSB has shown that proactive early intervention embedded in the principles of trauma-informed care is much more effective than a purely criminal justice or social care approach, especially if the child does not meet the criteria for a full AIM assessment and requires a more tailored response which offers help and support for parents or carers (Mercer, 2022).

Interventions with Siblings Who Have Experienced Sibling Sexual Abuse

Parental support is central in promoting better outcomes with regard to mental health and resolution of trauma (Caffaro, 2020; Yates & Allardyce, 2022). Professionals can facilitate parental support by emphasising the need to believe the child, validating the harm caused, providing emotional support, and by taking protective actions such as supervising interactions between the siblings. Parents will vary enormously with regard to their responses to SSA, how they conceptualise it and who they show their allegiance to, and who is the target for blame. Professionals will need to acknowledge this and take race, ethnicity, and cultural norms and expectations into consideration, and be mindful how these are reflected in family ideologies and identities.

Once disclosure has been made it is crucial to focus on resourcing the child who has been harmed and focus on their safety by ensuring that there is no escalation of SSA, or reprisals if the family remains intact. Children who have experienced SSA and later adult survivors need to be prioritised to access specialist trauma services that have experience of working with survivors of sexual abuse so that they can restore emotional regulation, manage trauma symptoms and dissociation, and process their experiences in a non-shaming, compassionate therapeutic environment (Tener et al., 2018 and Tener et al., 2020). It is also essential to take the feelings and concerns of the sibling who is being harmed into consideration if the sibling who has harmed remains in the family. McCartan et al. (2021) report that there is significant variation in adult survivors with regard to feeling safe when the sibling who has harmed remained in the family, as they lived in constant fear, while some preferred to keep the family intact as long as adequate supervision and reparative family therapy was in place.

Concluding Comments

To develop adequate protection and prevention takes time, resources, and effort, and needs to be supported by more research, national guidelines, policy changes, clear intervention protocols, psychoeducation, and training. Being able to access accurate information and knowledge will lead to changes in attitudes and beliefs about the normalisation of SSA, as well as making it easier for children to disclose, and families to respond appropriately. Society can also help with this by being more aware and not minimising the harmful effects of SSA or vilifying dual status children who commit SSA by seeing them as mini-adult sex offenders. Parents, adults, teachers, and professionals need to be empowered so that they can empower children and siblings to give voice to their experiences.

In order to prevent the sexual harm of children, whether through CSA, HSB, or SSA, we need to ensure that they are safe so that they can grow into healthy adults who are able to connect to others and flourish in their relationships. This is best facilitated through awareness that while many sibling relationships are positive and growth promoting, some are not safe and can cause physical, emotional, and sexual harm, and that subtle yet intrinsic power imbalances can lead to SSA. Equally, children can be equipped to be more aware of appropriate sexual behaviour by adults offering open communication, listening to their concerns, and ensuring that they are heard. We need to talk to them and educate them about safe touch, boundaries, and feeling safe. This includes guidance around respect, healthy boundaries, and consent, as well as the impact of early exposure to pornography.

To fully protect children, and help them and adult survivors to heal and recover from SSA, they need to be given a voice, be heard and believed rather than dismissed. This will enable them to feel safe in relationships where they can trust rather than fear, and fully connect to themselves and others.

Further Reading

Allardyce, S., & Yates, P. (2018). *Working with children and young people who have displayed harmful sexual behaviour.* Dunedin.

Caffaro, J. (2020). Sibling abuse of other children. In R. Geffner, V. Vieth, V. Vaughan-Eden, A. Rosenbaum, L. Hamberger, & J. White (eds), *Handbook of Interpersonal Violence across the Lifespan.* Springer.

Caffaro, J.V., & Conn-Caffaro, A. (1998). *Sibling abuse trauma: Assessment and intervention strategies for children, families and adults.* Routledge.

Hackett, S., Balfe, M., Masson, H., & Phillips, J. (2014). Family responses to young people who have sexually abused: Anger, ambivalence and acceptance. *Children & Society*, 28(2), 128–139.

McCartan, K., Anning, A., & Qureshi, E. (2021). *The impact of sibling sexual abuse on adults who were harmed as children.* UWE, Bristol Research Report.

Sanderson, C. (2004). *The seduction of children: Empowering parents and teachers to protect children from sexual abuse.* Jessica Kingsley Publishers.

Sanderson, C. (2022). *The warrior within: A One in Four handbook to aid recovery for survivors of childhood sexual abuse and violence* (4th edn). One in Four.

Yates, P., & Allardyce, S. (2021). *Sibling sexual abuse: Knowledge and practice.* Centre of Expertise on Child Sexual Abuse.

Yates, P., & Allardyce, S. (2022). Young people who sexually harm others. In R. Clawson, R. Fryson, & L. Warwick (eds), *The Child Protection Handbook* (4th edn). Elsevier.

References

Adler, N.A. & Schutz, J. (1995). Sibling incest offenders. *Child Abuse & Neglect, 19*(7), 811–819.
Allardyce, S., & Yates, P. (2013). Assessing risk of victim crossover in children and young people who display harmful sexual behaviours. *Child Abuse Review, 22*(4), 255–267.
Allardyce, S., & Yates, P. (2018). *Working with children and young people who have displayed harmful sexual behaviour.* Dunedin.
American Psychiatric Association. (2013). *Diagnostic and statistical manual of mental disorders: DSM-5* (Vol. 5). American Psychiatric Association.
Atwood, J.D. (2007). When love hurts: Preadolescent girls' reports of incest. *The American Journal of Family Therapy, 35*(4), 287–313.
Baldwin, J.D., & Baldwin, J.I. (2012). Sexual behaviour. In V. Ramachandran (ed.), *Encyclopedia of Human Behaviour* (2nd edn). Academic Press.
Ballantine, M.W. (2012). Sibling incest dynamics: Therapeutic themes and clinical challenges. *Clinical Social Work Journal, 40*(1), 56–65.
Baranowsky, A., & Gentry, J.E. (2014). *Trauma practice: Tools for stabilization and recovery.* Hogrefe Publishing.
Barra, S., Bessler, C., Landolt, M.A., & Aebi, M. (2018). Patterns of adverse childhood experiences in juveniles who sexually offended. *Sexual Abuse, 30*(7), 803–827.
Beckett, R. (2006). Risk prediction, decision making and evaluation of adolescent sexual abusers. In M. Erooga, & H. Masson (eds), *Children and young people who sexually abuse others* (2nd edn). Routledge.
Bentovim, A., Cox, A., Bingley-Miller, L., & Pizzey, S. (2009). *Safeguarding, living with trauma and family violence: A guide to evidence based analysis, planning and intervention.* Jessica Kingsley Publishing.
Berger, R., & Quiros, L. (2014). Supervision for trauma-informed practice. *Traumatology, 20*(4), 296.
Blue Seat Studios. (2015). Tea consent (clean). www.youtube.com/watch?v=fGoWLWS4-kU
Boon, S., Steele, K., & van der Hart, O. (2011). *Coping with trauma-related dissociation: Skills training for patients and therapists.* W.W. Norton.
Bovarnick, S., & Scott, S. (2016). *Child sexual exploitation prevention education: A rapid evidence assessment.* University of Bedfordshire.
Bowlby, J. (1973). *Attachment and loss*: Vol. 2. *Separation: Anxiety and anger.* Basic Books.
Boyle, M., & Johnstone, L. (2020). *A straight talking introduction to the Power Threat Meaning Framework: An alternative to psychiatric diagnosis.* PCCS Books.
Butler, L.D., Critelli, F.M., & Rinfrette, E.S. (2011). Trauma-informed care and mental health. *Directions in Psychiatry, 31*(3), 197–212.
Caffaro, J.V. (2017). Treating adult survivors of sibling sexual abuse: A relational strengths approach. *Journal of Family Violence, 32*, 543–552.

References

Caffaro, J.V. (2020). Sexual abuse of siblings. In T.K. Shackelford (ed.), *The SAGE Handbook of Domestic Violence*. SAGE.

Caffaro, J.V., & Conn-Caffaro, A. (1998). *Sibling abuse trauma: Assessment and intervention strategies for children, families and adults*. Routledge.

Caffaro, J.V., & Conn-Caffaro, A. (2014). *Sibling sexual trauma: Assessment and intervention, strategies for children, families and adults*. Routledge.

Campbell, S.M. (2016). The concept of well-being. In G. Fletcher (ed.), *The Routledge handbook of philosophy of well-being*. Routledge.

Canavan, M.M., Meyer III, W.J., & Higgs, D.C. (1992). The female experience of sibling incest. *Journal of Marital and Family Therapy*, 18(2), 129–142.

Carlson, B.E., Maciol, K., & Schneider, J. (2006). Sibling incest: Reports from forty-one survivors. *Journal of Child Sexual Abuse*, 15(4), 19–34.

Caspi, J. (2011). *Sibling aggression: Assessment and treatment*. Springer.

Choi, K.R., Seng, J.S., Briggs, E.C., Munro-Kramer, M.L., Graham-Bermann, S.A., Lee, R., & Ford, J.D. (2018). *Dissociation and PTSD: What parents should know*. National Center for Child Traumatic Stress.

Cloitre, M., Courtois, C.A., Ford, J.D., Green, B.L., Alexander, P., Briere, J., & Van der Hart, O. (2012). The ISTSS expert consensus treatment guidelines for complex PTSD in adults. ISTSS. https://istss.org/ISTSS_Main/media/Documents/ComplexPTSD.pdf

Cohen, J.A., & Scheeringa, M.S. (2009). Post-traumatic stress disorder diagnosis in children: Challenges and promises. *Dialogues in Clinical Neuroscience*, 11(1), 91–99.

Courtois, C.A., & Ford, J.D. (2012). *Treatment of complex trauma: A sequenced, relationship-based approach*. Guilford Press.

Cozolino, L. (2021). *The development of a therapist: Healing others – healing self* (Kindle edn). W.W. Norton.

Cundy, L. (2015). Attachment, self-experience, and communication technology: Love in the age of the internet. In *Love in the age of the internet: Attachment in the digital era*. Routledge.

Cyr, M., Wright, J., McDuff, P., & Perron, A. (2002). Intrafamilial sexual abuse: Brother–sister incest does not differ from father–daughter and stepfather–stepdaughter incest. *Child Abuse and Neglect*, 26, 957–973.

De Jong, A.R. (1989). Sexual interactions among siblings and cousins: Experimentation or exploitation? *Child Abuse & Neglect*, 13(2), 271–279.

Department for Education. (2018). *Working together to safeguard children: A guide to inter-agency working to safeguard and promote the welfare of children*. DfE.

Department of Health. (2000). *Framework for the assessment of children in need and their families*. The Stationery Office.

DiGiorgio-Miller, J. (1998). Sibling incest: Treatment of the family and the offender. *Child Welfare*, 77(3), 335–346.

Elliott, D.E., Bjelajac, P., Fallot, R.D., Markoff, L.S., & Reed, B.G. (2005). Trauma-informed or trauma-denied: Principles and implementation of trauma-informed services for women. *Journal of Community Psychology*, 33(4), 461–477.

Enns, C.Z., McNeilly, C.L., Corkery, J.M., & Gilbert, M.S. (1995). The debate about delayed memories of child sexual abuse: A feminist perspective. *The Counseling Psychologist*, 23(2), 181–279.

Erooga, M., & Masson, H. (2006). *Children and young people who sexually abuse others: Current developments and practice responses* (2nd edn). Routledge.

Fallot, R.D., & Harris, M. (2008). Trauma-informed approaches to systems of care. *Trauma Psychology Newsletter*, 3(1), 6–7.

Felitti, V.J., Anda, R.F., Nordenberg, D., & Williamson, D.F. (1998). Adverse childhood experiences and health outcomes in adults: The Ace study. *Journal of Family and Consumer Sciences*, 90(3), 31.

Finkelhor, D. (2009). *Children's exposure to violence: A comprehensive national survey*. Diane Publishing.

Finkelhor, D., Hotaling, G., Lewis, I., & Smith, C. (1989). Sexual abuse and its relationship to later sexual satisfaction, marital status, religion and attitudes. *Journal of Interpersonal Violence, 4*(4), 379–399.

Fisher, J. (2021). *Transforming the living legacy of trauma: A workbook for survivors and therapists*. PESI.

Fonagy, P., & Adshead, G. (2012). How mentalisation changes the mind. *Advances in Psychiatric Treatment, 18*(5), 353–362.

Ford, J.D., Courtois, C.A., Steele, K., Hart, O.V.D., & Nijenhuis, E.R. (2005). Treatment of complex posttraumatic self-dysregulation. *Journal of Traumatic Stress: Official Publication of the International Society for Traumatic Stress Studies, 18*(5), 437–447.

Forgash, C., & Knipe, J. (2008). Integrating EMDR and ego state therapy for client with trauma disorder. In C.L. Forgash, & M. Copeley (eds), *Healing the heart of trauma and dissociation with EMDR and ego state therapy*. Springer.

Frawley, P., & Wilson, N.J. (2016). Young people with intellectual disability talking about sexuality education and information. *Sexuality and Disability, 34*, 469–484.

Friedrich, W., Fisher, J., Broughton, D., Houston, M., & Shafran, C. (1998). Normative sexual behaviour in children: A contemporary sample. *Pediatrics, 101*(4), e9.

Gelinas, D.J. (2003). Integrating EMDR into phase-oriented treatment for trauma. *Journal of Trauma & Dissociation, 4*(3), 91–135.

Glaser, D. (1991). Treatment issues in child sexual abuse. *The British Journal of Psychiatry, 159*(6), 769–782.

Griffee, K., Swindell, S., O'Keefe, S.L., Stroebel, S.S., Beard, K.W., Kuo, S.-Y., & Stroupe, W. (2016). Etiological risk factors for sibling incest: Data from an anonymous computer-assisted self-interview. *Sexual Abuse: Journal of Research and Treatment, 28*(7), 620–659.

Hackett, S. (2001). *Facing the future: A guide for parents of young people who have sexually abused*. Russell House Publishing.

Hackett, S. (2004). *What works for children and young people with harmful sexual behaviours?* Barnardo's.

Hackett, S. (2010). Children and young people with harmful sexual behaviours. In C. Barter, & D. Berridge (eds), *Children behaving badly? Peer violence between children and young people*. Wiley-Blackwell.

Hackett, S. (2014). *Children and young people with harmful sexual behaviours: Research review*. Research in Practice.

Hackett, S., Balfe, M., Masson, H., & Phillips, J. (2014). Family responses to young people who have sexually abused: Anger, ambivalence and acceptance. *Children & Society, 28*(2), 128–139.

Hackett, S., Branigan, P., & Holmes, D. (2019). *Harmful sexual behaviour framework: An evidence-informed operational framework for children and young people displaying harmful sexual behaviours* (2nd edn). NSPCC.

Hackett, S., Phillips, J., Masson, H., & Balfe, M. (2013). Individual, family and abuse characteristics of 700 British child and adolescent sexual abusers. *Child Abuse Review, 22*(4), 232–245.

Hardy, M.S. (2001). Physical aggression and sexual behavior among siblings: A retrospective study. *Journal of Family Violence, 16*, 255–268.

Herman, J.L. (1992). Complex PTSD: A syndrome in survivors of prolonged and repeated trauma. *Journal of Traumatic Stress, 5*(3), 377–391.

Herman, J.L. (2001). *Trauma and recovery* (2nd edn). Basic Books.

Herman, J.L. (2015). *Trauma and recovery: The aftermath of violence – From domestic abuse to political terror*. Hachette UK.

Herman, J.L. (2023). *Truth and repair: How trauma survivors envision justice*. Basic Books.

Hollis, V., & Belton, E. (2017). *Children and young people who engage in technology-assisted harmful sexual behaviour*. NSPCC.

Howell, E.F. (2011). *Understanding and treating dissociative identity disorder*. Routledge.

Howell, E.F. (2013). *The dissociative mind*. Routledge.

International Society for the Study of Trauma and Dissociation. (2011). Guidelines for treating dissociative identity disorder in adults, third revision. *Journal of Trauma & Dissociation*, *12*(2), 115–187.

Johnson, T. (2015). *Understanding children's sexual behaviors – What's natural and healthy* (expanded edn). Neari Press.

Johnstone, L., & Boyle, M. with Cromby, J., Dillon, J., Harper, D., Kinderman, P., Longden, E., Pilgrim, D., & Read, J. (2018). *The Power Threat Meaning Framework: Towards the identification of patterns in emotional distress, unusual experiences and troubled or troubling behaviour, as an alternative to functional psychiatric diagnosis*. British Psychological Society.

Jordan, J.V. (2000). The role of mutual empathy in relational/cultural therapy. *Journal of Clinical Psychology*, *56*(8), 1005–1016.

Jordan, J.V. (2017). Relational-cultural theory: The power of connection to transform our lives. *The Journal of Humanistic Counselling*, *56*, 3.

Katz, C., & Hamama, L. (2017). From my own brother in my own home: Children's experiences and perceptions following alleged sibling familial sexual abuse. *Journal of Child Sexual Abuse*, *32*(23), 3648–3668.

Kelly, L. (1992). The connections between disability and child abuse: A review of the research evidence. *Child Abuse Review*, *1*(3), 157–167.

Khantzian, E.J., & Albanese, M.J. (2008). *Understanding addiction as self-medication: Finding hope behind the pain*. Rowman & Littlefield Publishers.

Krienert, J.L., & Walsh, J.A. (2011). Sibling sexual abuse: An empirical analysis of offender, victim, and event characteristics in national incident-based reporting system (NIBRS) data, 2000–2007. *Journal of Child Sexual Abuse*, *20*, 353–372.

Lanius, R.A., Terpou, B.A., & McKinnon, M.C. (2020). The sense of self in the aftermath of trauma: Lessons from the default mode network in posttraumatic stress disorder. *European Journal of Psychotraumatology*, *11*(1), 1807703.

Latzman, N.E., Viljoen, J.L., Scalora, M.J., & Ullman, D. (2011). Sexual offending in adolescence: A comparison of sibling offenders and nonsibling offenders across domains of risk and treatment need. *Journal of Child Sexual Abuse*, *20*(3), 245–263.

Laviola, M. (1992). Effects of older brother-younger sister incest: A study of the dynamics of 17 cases. *Child Abuse & Neglect*, *16*(3), 409–421.

Letourneau, E.J., Schaeffer, C.M., Bradshaw, C.P., & Feder, K.A. (2017). Preventing the onset of child sexual abuse by targeting young adolescents with universal prevention programming. *Child Maltreatment*, *22*(2), 100–111.

Levine, P.A. (1997). *Waking the tiger*. North Atlantic Books.

Lewis, H.B. (1971). *Shame and guilt in neurosis*. International Universities Press.

Loredo, C. (1982). Sibling incest. In S. Sgroi (ed.), *Handbook of clinical intervention in child sexual abuse*. Free Press.

Lussier, P., & Blokland, A. (2014). The adolescence-adulthood transition and Robins's continuity paradox: Criminal career patterns of juvenile and adult sex offenders in a prospective longitudinal birth cohort study. *Journal of Criminal Justice*, *42*, 153–163.

Maltsberger, J.T., & Buie, D.H. (1974). Countertransference hate in the treatment of suicidal patients. *Archives of General Psychiatry*, *30*(5), 625–633.

Masson, H., & Hackett, S. (2003). A decade on from the NCH Report (1992): Adolescent sexual aggression policy, practice and service delivery across the UK and Republic of Ireland. *Journal of Sexual Aggression*, *9*(2), 109–124.

Maté, G. (2009). *In the realm of hungry ghosts: Close encounters with addiction*. Vintage Canada.

McCartan, K., Anning, A., & Qureshi, E. (2021). *The impact of sibling sexual abuse on adults who were harmed as children*. UWE, Bristol Research Report.

McKillop, N., Brown, S., Smallbone, S., & Pritchard, K. (2015). Similarities and differences in adolescence-onset versus adulthood-onset sexual abuse incidents. *Child Abuse & Neglect, 46*, 37–46.

McNeish, D., & Scott, S. (2018). *Key messages from research on intra-familial child sexual abuse*. Centre of Expertise on Child Sexual Abuse.

Mead, D., & Sharpe, M. (2017). Pornography and sexuality research papers at the 4th International Conference on Behavioral Addictions. *Sexual Addiction & Compulsivity: The Journal of Treatment & Prevention, 24*(3), 217–223.

Mercer, J. (2022). Critiquing assumptions about parental alienation: Part 2. Causes of psychological harms. *Journal of Family Trauma, Child Custody & Child Development, 19*(2), 139–156.

Miller, J.B. (2015). *The healing connection: How women form relationships in therapy and in life*. Beacon Press.

Mollon, P. (2000). Dissociative identity disorder. In C.A. Hooper, & U. McCluskey (eds), *Psychodynamic perspectives on abuse: The cost of fear*. Jessica Kingsley Publishers.

Najavits, L. (2002). *Seeking safety: A treatment manual for PTSD and substance abuse*. Guilford Press.

Nathanson, D.L. (1992). *Shame and pride: Affect, sex, and the birth of the self*. W.W. Norton.

NSPCC. (2003). *Annual report: Someone to turn to for every child*. NSPCC.

NSPCC. (2021). *Statistics briefing: Sexual harmful behaviour*. NSPCC.

Ogden, P. (2015). *Sensorimotor psychotherapy*. W.W. Norton.

Ogden, P., Minton, K., & Pain, C. (2006). *Trauma and the body: A sensorimotor approach to psychotherapy* (Norton series on interpersonal neurobiology). W.W. Norton.

O'Brien, M.J. (1991). Taking sibling incest seriously. In M.Q. Patton (ed.), *Family sexual abuse: Frontline research and evaluation*. SAGE.

O'Keefe, S.L., Beard, K.W., Swindell, S., Stroebel, S.S., Griffee, K., & Young, D.H. (2014). Sister–brother incest: Data from anonymous computer assisted self-interviews. *Sexual Addiction and Compulsivity: The Journal of Treatment and Prevention, 21*(1), 1–38.

One in Four. (2015). *Survivors' voices*. One in Four.

One in Four. (2019). *Numbing the pain*. One in Four.

Payne, P., Levine, P.A., & Crane-Godreau, M.A. (2015). Somatic experiencing: Using interoception and proprioception as core elements of trauma therapy. *Frontiers in Psychology, 6*, 93.

Perry, B.D. (2019). The neurosequential model. In J. Mitchell, J. Tucci, & E. Tronick (eds), *The handbook of therapeutic care for children: Evidence-informed approaches to working with traumatized children and adolescents in foster, kinship and adoptive care*. Jessica Kingsley Publishers.

Punch, S. (2008). 'You can do nasty things to your brothers and sisters without a reason': Siblings' backstage behaviour. *Children & Society, 22*(5), 333–344.

Putnam, F.W. (1993). Dissociative disorders in children: Behavioural profiles and problems. *Child Abuse & Neglect, 17*(1), 39–45.

Quiros, L., & Berger, R. (2015). Responding to the socio-political complexity of trauma: An integration of theory and practice. *Journal of Loss and Trauma, 20*(2), 149–159.

Rothschild, B. (2000). *The body remembers: The psychophysiology of trauma and trauma treatment*. W.W. Norton & Company.

Rothschild, B. (2017). *The body remembers. Volume 2: Revolutionizing trauma treatment*. W.W. Norton.

Rothschild, B. (2021). *Revolutionizing trauma treatment: Stabilization, safety, & nervous system balance*. W.W. Norton.

Ryan, G. (2000). Childhood sexuality: A decade of study. Part I – Research and curriculum development. *Child Abuse & Neglect, 24*(1), 33–48.

Saakvitne, K.W., & Pearlman, L.A. (1996). *Transforming the pain: A workbook on vicarious traumatization*. W.W. Norton.

Sabina, C., Wolak, J., & Finkelhor, D. (2008). The nature and dynamics of internet pornography exposure for youth. *CyberPsychology & Behavior, 11*(6), 691–693.

Sanderson, C. (2004). *The seduction of children: Empowering parents and teachers to protect children from sexual abuse*. Jessica Kingsley Publishers.

Sanderson, C. (2006). *Counselling adult survivors of child sexual abuse* (3rd edn). Jessica Kingsley Publishers.

Sanderson, C. (2013). *Counselling skills for working with trauma*. Jessica Kingsley Publishers.

Sanderson, C. (2015). *Counselling skills for working with shame*. Jessica Kingsley Publishers.

Sanderson, C. (2016). *The warrior within: A One in Four handbook to aid recovery for survivors*. One in Four.

Sanderson, C. (2017). *Dissociation and dissociative disorders: Advice for adults suffering with dissociation and those working with them*. One in Four.

Sanderson, C. (2019). *Numbing the pain: A pocket guide for professionals supporting survivors of childhood sexual abuse and addiction*. One in Four.

Sanderson, C. (2022). *The warrior within: A One in Four handbook to aid recovery for survivors of childhood sexual abuse and violence* (4th edn). One in Four.

Saunders, B., Berliner, L., & Hanson, R. (eds) (2003) *Child physical and sexual abuse: Guidelines for treatment*. Final report: January 15, 2003. National Crime Victims Research and Treatment Center.

Scheeringa, M.S. (2011). PTSD in children younger than the age of 13: Toward developmentally sensitive assessment and management. *Journal of Child & Adolescent Trauma, 4*, 181–197.

Schimmenti, A., & Caretti, V. (2016). Linking the overwhelming with the unbearable: Developmental trauma, dissociation, and the disconnected self. *Psychoanalytic Psychology, 33*(1), 106.

Shah, R.S. (2017). How sex offender registries impact youth. *Teen Vogue: Kids Incarcerated*. www.teenvogue.com/story/how-sex-offender-registries-impact-youth

Shapiro, E. (2009). EMDR treatment of recent trauma. *Journal of EMDR Practice and Research, 3*(3), 141–151.

Shaw, J.A., Lewis, J.E., Loeb, A., Rosado, J., & Rodriguez, R.A. (2000). Child on child sexual abuse: Psychological perspectives. *Child Abuse & Neglect, 24*(12), 1591–1600.

Shonkoff, J.P., & Bales, S.N. (2011). Science does not speak for itself: Translating child development research for the public and its policymakers. *Child Development, 82*(1), 17–32.

Siegel, D.J. (1999). *The developing mind: Toward a neurobiology of interpersonal experience*. Guilford Press.

Skovholt, T.M., & Trotter-Mathison, M. (2016). *The resilient practitioner: Burnout and compassion fatigue prevention and self-care strategies for the helping professions*. Routledge.

Smith, C., Bradbury-Jones, C., Lazenbatt, A., & Taylor, J. (2013). *Provision for young people who have displayed harmful sexual behaviour: An understanding of contemporary service provision for young people displaying harmful sexual behaviour in a UK context*. NSPCC.

Smith, C., Allardyce, S., Hackett, S., Bradbury-Jones, C., Lazenbatt, A., & Taylor, J. (2014). Practice and policy in the UK with children and young people who display harmful sexual behaviour: An analysis and critical review. *Journal of Sexual Aggression, 20*(3), 267–280.

Smith, H., & Israel, E. (1987). Sibling incest: A study of the dynamics of 25 cases. *Child Abuse & Neglect, 11*(1), 101–108.

Spinazzola, J., Van der Kolk, B., & Ford, J.D. (2021). Developmental trauma disorder: A legacy of attachment trauma in victimized children. *Journal of Traumatic Stress, 34*(4), 711–720.

Stathopoulos, M. (2012). Sibling sexual abuse. www.decision-making-confidence.com/support-files/australian-institute-of-family-studies

Steele, K., & Van der Hart, O. (2009). Treating dissociation. In C.A. Courtois & J.D. Ford (eds), *Treating complex traumatic stress disorders: An evidence-based guide*. Guilford Press.

Steele, K., Boon, S., & Van der Hart, O. (2017). *Treating trauma related dissociation: A practical, integrative approach*. W.W. Norton.

Stripe, T.S., & Stermac, L.E. (2003). An exploration of childhood victimization and family-of-origin characteristics of sexual offenders against children. *International Journal of Offender Therapy and Comparative Criminology, 47*(5), 542–555.

Stroebel, S.S., O'Keefe, S.L., Beard, K.W., Kuo, S.-Y., Swindell, S., & Stroupe, W. (2013). Brother–sister incest: Data from anonymous computer-assisted self-interviews. *Journal of Child Sexual Abuse, 22*(3), 255–276.

Tangney, J.P., & Dearing, R.L. (2002). *Shame and guilt*. Guilford Press.

Tener, D. (2019). 'I love and hate him in the same breath': Relationships of adult survivors of sexual abuse with their perpetrating siblings. *Journal of Interpersonal Violence, 36*(13–14), NP6844–NP6866.

Tener, D., Katz, C., & Kaufmann, Y. (2020). 'And I let it all out': Survivors' sibling sexual abuse disclosures. *Journal of Interpersonal Violence, 36*(23–24), 11140–11164.

Tener, D., Lusky, E., Tarshish, N., & Turjeman, S. (2018). Parental attitudes following disclosure of sibling sexual abuse: A child advocacy centre intervention study. *American Journal of Orthopsychiatry, 88*(6), 661–669.

Tener, D., Tarshish, N., & Turgeman, S. (2017). 'Victim, perpetrator, or just my brother?' Sibling sexual abuse in large families: A child advocacy centre study. *Journal of Interpersonal Violence, 35*(21–22), 4887–4912.

Tidefors, I., Arvidsson, H., Ingevaldson, S., & Larsson, M. (2010). Sibling incest: A literature review and a clinical study. *Journal of Sexual Aggression, 16*(3), 347–360.

Tougas, A.M., Boisvert, I., Tourigny, M., Lemieux, A., Tremblay, C., & Gagnon, M.M. (2016). Psychosocial profile of children having participated in an intervention program for their sexual behavior problems: The predictor role of maltreatment. *Journal of Child Sexual Abuse, 25*(2), 127–141.

Turner, H.A., Finkelhor, D., & Ormrod, R. (2010). Poly-victimization in a national sample of children and youth. *American Journal of Preventive Medicine, 38*(3), 323–330.

Twombly, J.H. (2005). EMDR for clients with dissociative identity disorder, DDNOS, and ego states. In R. Shapiro (ed.), *EMDR solutions: Pathways to healing*. W.W. Norton.

Van der Hart, O., & Rydberg, J.A. (2019). Vehement emotions and trauma-related dissociation: A Janetian perspective on integrative failure. *European Journal of Trauma and Dissociation, 3*(3), 191–201.

Van der Hart, O., Nijenhuis, E.R., & Steele, K. (2006). *The haunted self: Structural dissociation and the treatment of chronic traumatization*. W.W. Norton.

Van der Hart, O., Nijenhuis, E., Steele, K., & Brown, D. (2004). Trauma-related dissociation: Conceptual clarity lost and found. *Australian & New Zealand Journal of Psychiatry*, *38*(11-12), 906–914.

Van der Kolk, B. (2015). *The body keeps the score: Mind, brain and body in the transformation of trauma*. Penguin Books.

Van der Kolk, B., Ford, J.D., & Spinazzola, J. (2019). Comorbidity of developmental trauma disorder (DTD) and post-traumatic stress disorder: Findings from the DTD field trial. *European Journal of Psychotraumatology*, *10*(1), 1562841.

Veale, D., Freeston, M., Krebs, G., Heyman, I., & Salkovskis, P. (2009). Risk assessment and management in obsessive–compulsive disorder. *Advances in Psychiatric Treatment*, *15*(5), 332–343.

Vizard, E., Hickey, N., French, L., & McCrory, E. (2007). Children and adolescents who present with sexually abusive behaviour: A UK descriptive study. *The Journal of Forensic Psychiatry & Psychology*, *18*(1), 59–73.

Ward, T. (2002). The management of risk and the design of good lives. *Australian Psychologist*, *37*(3), 172–179.

Ward, T., Mann, R., & Gannon, T. (2007). The good lives model of offender rehabilitation: Clinical implications. *Aggression and Violent Behavior*, *12*(1), 87–107.

White, N., & Hughes, C. (2018). *Why siblings matter: The role of brother and sister relationships in development and well-being*. Routledge.

Wiehe, V.R. (1997). *Sibling abuse: Hidden physical, emotional, and sexual trauma*. SAGE.

Wiehe, V.R. (1998). *Understanding family violence: Treating and preventing partner, child, sibling and elder abuse*. SAGE.

Wissink, I.B., Van Vugt, E., Moonen, X., Stams, G.J.J., & Hendriks, J. (2015). Sexual abuse involving children with an intellectual disability (ID): A narrative review. *Research in Developmental Disabilities*, *36*, 20–35.

World Health Organization. (2018). ICD-11 for mortality and morbidity statistics. WHO. https://icd.who.int/browse/11/2018/mms/en

Worling, J.R. (1995). Adolescent sibling-incest offenders: Differences in family and individual functioning when compared to adolescent nonsibling sex offenders. *Child Abuse & Neglect*, *19*(5), 633–643.

Yates, P. (2017). Sibling sexual abuse: Why don't we talk about it? *Journal of Clinical Nursing*, *26*(15–16), 2482–2494.

Yates, P. (2018). 'Siblings as better together': Social worker decision-making in cases involving sibling sexual behaviour. *British Journal of Social Work*, *48*(1), 176–194.

Yates, P. (2020). 'It's just the abuse that needs to stop': Professional framing of sibling relationships in a grounded theory study of social worker decision-making following sibling abuse. *Journal of Child Sexual Abuse*, *29*(2), 222–245.

Yates, P., & Allardyce, S. (2021). *Sibling sexual abuse: Knowledge and practice*. Centre of Expertise on Child Sexual Abuse.

Yates, P., & Allardyce, S. (2022). Abuse at the heart of the family: The challenges and complexities of sibling sexual abuse. In K. Uzieblo, W.J. Smid, & K. McCartan (eds), *Challenges in the Management of People Convicted of a Sexual Offence*. Palgrave Macmillan.

Yates, P., Allardyce, S., & MacQueen, S. (2012). Children who display harmful sexual behaviour: Assessing the risks of boys abusing at home, in the community or across both settings. *Journal of Sexual Aggression*, *18*(1), 23–35.

Resources

One in Four
Advocacy, counselling and information for people who have experienced sexual abuse.

> Telephone 020 8697 2112
> Email admin@oneinfour.org.uk
> www.oneinfour.org.uk

Childline
A free and confidential helpline for children and young adults in the UK. It offers help and advice plus volunteering and fundraising details. Secure messages can be sent via their website.

> Freephone helplines (24hr) – children 0800 1111; parents and professionals 0808 800 5000
> Email via the website www.childline.org.uk

Everyone's Invited
A safe place for survivors to share their stories online completely anonymously. The act of sharing their story allows many survivors a sense of relief, catharsis, empowerment, and gives them a feeling of community and hope.

> www.everyonesinvited.uk

Family Matters
Counselling service in Kent for children and adult survivors of sexual abuse and rape.

> Telephone 01474 536 661
> Helpline 01474 537 392
> Email admin@familymattersuk.org
> www.familymattersuk.org

#SiblingsToo
#SiblingsToo aim to break the silence of sibling sexual abuse with real science and heartfelt stories so that society is empowered (and even compelled) to do something about it. They aim to do this using the #SiblingsToo podcast series (https://siblingstoo.libsyn.com/) as well as the story-gathering tool used on this site. By anonymously sharing your story of SSA, whether as the survivor, perpetrator, or any member of the family, you will be speaking volumes to the rest of society while also helping researchers and experts understand more about the prevalence and impacts of SSA.

Sibling Sexual Abuse Project
Support helpline for adults and young people aged 13+. Their helpline is open to all: adults and young people aged 13+ of all genders can get in contact for support.

>Helpline 0808 801 0456 (open Monday: 11am–2pm; Tuesday: 6pm–8pm; Wednesday: 6pm–8pm; Thursday: 6pm–8pm; Friday: 11am–2pm)
>Email support@sarsas.org.uk

Phone one of the helplines that follow in this section or contact the following agencies if you suspect a child is being abused or is at risk of abuse, or you know of an abuser who has any contact with children.

Police
Many districts now have a special police unit that works with sexual abuse. Phone your local police station and ask to speak to the officer who deals with sexual abuse.

Social services
Phone your local office and ask for the child protection officer or the duty officer.

If you are abusing children or have urges to abuse children contact the NSPCC, social services, or the police.

HAVOCA (Help for Adult Victims of Child Abuse)
Provides information to any adult who is suffering from past childhood abuse. Website includes survivors' forum.

>Email via the website www.havoca.org

Kidscape
Kidscape produces leaflets and booklets on bullying, and runs a helpline.

>Parent advice line 020 7823 5430 (Monday and Tuesday 9.30am–2.30pm)
>Email (parent support) parentsupport@kidscape.org.uk; (general enquiries) info@kidscape.org.uk www.kidscape.org.uk

Lifecentre
Telephone counselling for survivors of sexual abuse and those supporting them. Face-to-face counselling and art therapy groups in West Sussex.

>Helpline 0808 802 0808 (Sunday, Monday, Tuesday, and Thursday 7.30–10pm)
>Text 07717 989 022
>Email via website www.lifecentre.uk.com

National Association of People Abused in Childhood (NAPAC)
A UK charity providing support and information for people abused in childhood.

>Freephone helpline 0808 801 0331 (Monday to Thursday 10am–9pm, Friday 10am–6pm)
>Email support@napac.org.uk
>www.napac.org.uk

National Society for Prevention of Cruelty to Children (NSPCC)
Works to end cruelty to children in the UK by standing up for their rights, listening to them, helping them, and making them safe. Free 24hr national helpline for information and confidential advice about all types of problems.

> Helpline 0808 800 5000 (Monday to Friday 8am–10pm, Saturday and Sunday 9am–6pm)
> Email help@nspcc.org.uk
> www.nspcc.org.uk

Rape and Sexual Abuse Support Centre (RASASC)
National helpline for female and male survivors, partners, friends, and family.

> Freephone helpline 0808 802 9999 (12–2.30pm and 7–9.30pm daily)
> Email info@rasasc.org.uk
> www.rasasc.org.uk

Survivors in Transition (SiT)
A support centre based in Suffolk offering counselling, information, advice, guidance, and referrals to other specialist organisations for men and women who have experienced any form of CSA.

> Telephone 07765 052282 or 01473 232499
> Email support@survivorsintransition.co.uk
> www.survivorsintransition.co.uk

The Survivors Trust
A national umbrella agency for 130 specialist voluntary sector agencies that provide a range of counselling, therapeutic, and support services.

> Helpline 0808 801 0818 (Monday to Thursday 10am–12.30pm, 1.30pm–5.30pm, and 6pm–8pm; Friday 10am–12.30pm and 1.30pm–5.30pm; Saturday 10am–1pm; Sunday 5pm–8pm)
> Email info@thesurvivorstrust.org
> www.thesurvivorstrust.org

Support for Women
CIS'ters (Childhood Incest Survivors)
Based in Hampshire, providing help and support for adult women who suffered incest as a child. Organises workshops and conferences to raise awareness on the issues surrounding incest, particularly mental distress.

> Telephone 023 8033 8080
> Email helpme@cisters.org.uk
> www.cisters.org.uk

Rape Crisis (England and Wales)
Lists local organisations across England and Wales with contact details, services offered, and opening times. Services are available to women who have been sexually abused at any time in their lives.

>National freephone helpline 0808 802 9999 (every day 12–12.30pm and 7–9.30pm)
Email rcewinfo@rapecrisis.org.uk
Live chat via the website www.rapecrisis.org.uk

Rights of Women
Based in London, informing, educating, and empowering women on their legal rights.

>Administration 020 7251 6575
National family law line 020 7251 6577 (Tuesday to Thursday 7–9pm, Friday 12–2pm)
London family law line 020 7608 1137 (Monday 10am–12pm and 2pm–4pm; Tuesday and Wednesday 2–4pm; and Thursday 10am–12pm and 2–4pm)
Email info@row.org.uk
www.rightsofwomen.org.uk

Solace Women's Aid
An independent charity providing a comprehensive range of services for women and children affected by domestic and sexual violence.

>Freephone helpline 0808 802 5565 (Monday 10am–4pm; Tuesday 6pm–8pm; Wednesday to Friday 10am–4pm)
Email advice@solacewomensaid.org
www.solacewomensaid.org

Women's Aid
A national charity working to end domestic violence against women and children.

>Email info@womensaid.org.uk
Live chat via chat.womensaid.org.uk
www.womensaid.org.uk

Women and Girls Network
Provides face-to-face counselling and support groups in the London area.

>Telephone 020 3598 3898
Email help@survivorsuk.org
Live chat via the website (Monday to Sunday 12–8pm) www.survivorsuk.org

Support for Non-Abusive Parents and Carers of Children Who Have Been Sexually Abused
Mosac
A charity supporting non-abusing parents and carers whose children have been sexually abused, providing them with support, advice, information, and counselling.

>Freephone helpline 0800 980 1958 (Monday to Friday, except bank holidays)
Email via the website www.mosac.org.uk

Support to Prevent Sexual Abuse of Children
Stop It Now!
Confidential help for people struggling with sexual thoughts and behaviours towards children. They will also support anyone with a concern, including the parents and carers of children and young people with worrying sexual behaviour, and friends and family worried about the behaviour of another adult.

>Freephone helpline 0808 1000 900 (Monday to Thursday 9am–9pm and Friday 9am–5pm)
>Email and live chat via the website www.stopitnow.org.uk

Women & Girls Network
Counselling, support, and advice for women who have been affected by gendered violence, including sexual and domestic violence.

>Freephone advice 0808 801 0660 (Monday to Friday 10am–4pm and Wednesday 6–9pm)
>Sexual violence helpline 0808 801 0770 (Monday and Friday 10am–12.30pm and 2.30–4.30pm; Wednesday 6–9pm)
>Email advice@wgn.org.uk
>www.wgn.org.uk

Women in Prison
A national charity based in London supporting women affected by the criminal justice system and campaigning for social justice.

>Telephone 020 7359 6674
>Email info@wipuk.org
>www.womeninprison.org.uk

Support for Men
ManKind Initiative
A helpline service for male victims of domestic abuse or domestic violence.

>Helpline 01823 334 244 (Monday to Friday 10am–4pm)
>www.mankind.org.uk

SurvivorsUK
Provides a national online helpline, individual and group counselling for boys, men, and non-binary people aged 13+ who have experienced sexual violence at any time in their lives. Also offers emotional support through the justice system, support for friends and families of survivors, and training for professionals and organisations. SurvivorsUK currently operates both remotely and in-person from their office and various venues across London.

>Telephone 02035983898
>Email help@survivorsuk.org
>www.survivorsuk.org

Specialist Therapy, Counselling, and Support

Action for Children
Based in Watford, providing a national network offering support and counselling for children and their families.

    Telephone 0300 123 2112 (Monday to Friday 9am–5pm)
    Email ask.us@actionforchildren.org.uk
    www.actionforchildren.org.uk

British Association for Counselling and Psychotherapy (BACP)
A professional body representing counselling and psychotherapy with over 40,000 members, working towards a better standard of therapeutic practice.

    Telephone 01455 883 300 (Monday to Friday 10am–4pm)
    Email bacp@bacp.co.uk
    www.bacp.co.uk
    Or visit the website of the British Psychological Society www.bps.org.uk

DABS (Directory and Book Services)
DABS collates information to produce a national directory for survivor resources.

    www.dabs.uk.com

EMDR Association
Information about EMDR (eye movement desensitisation and reprocessing) and help to find an accredited UK therapist.

    www.emdrassociation.org.uk

MIND
The leading mental health charity promoting understanding of mental health.

    Telephone 020 8519 2122
    Infoline 0300 123 3393 (Monday to Friday 9am–6pm)
    Email info@mind.org.uk
    www.mind.org.uk

Relate
A nationwide charity helping with relationship difficulties and sexual problems and providing couples counselling.

    Live chat, email, and contact details via the website www.relate.org.uk

Victim Support
A nationwide charity co-ordinating nationwide support schemes, dedicated to supporting victims of crime and traumatic incidents in England and Wales.

    Support line 0808 1689 111 (every day 24hr)
    www.victimsupport.org.uk

Children 1st
Scotland's national children's charity providing holistic family support and trauma recovery for children, young people, and their families.

> Telephone 0131 446 2300
> Children 1st Parentline 08000 28 22 33 (Monday to Friday 9am–9pm, Saturday and Sunday 9am–12pm)
> Email cfs@children1st.org.uk
> www.children1st.org.uk

Clinical psychologists
Your GP can refer you to a clinical psychologist or you can ask another professional for advice on how to get to see a psychologist.

Specialist Agencies
ACAL (Association of Child Abuse Lawyers)
Set up by leading solicitors in the field for the benefit of victims, survivors, lawyers, experts, and other professionals involved in obtaining compensation for the physical, sexual, or emotional abuse of children and adults abused in childhood.

> Telephone 020 8390 4701 (Tuesday and Thursday 10am–1pm and 2–4pm)
> Email via the website www.childabuselawyers.com

Ann Craft Trust (ACT)
An information and networking service for adult and child survivors with learning disabilities and workers involved in this area.

> Telephone 0115 951 5400
> Email ann-craft-trust@nottingham.ac.uk
> www.anncrafttrust.org

CICA (Criminal Injuries Compensation Authority)
CICA deal with compensation claims from people who have been physically or mentally injured because they were the victim of a violent crime in England, Scotland, or Wales.

> Telephone 0300 003 3601
> www.gov.uk/government/organisations/criminal-injuries-compensation-authority

Heal for Life Foundation UK
Based in Kent, providing residential healing programmes in Essex for survivors of CSA.

> Telephone 01233 813884
> Email admin@healforlife.org.uk
> www.healforlife.org.uk

Irwin Mitchell Solicitors
Offer help, advice and represent individuals in any area of law, including personal injury. Have represented and advocated on behalf of survivors of child sexual abuse.

>Telephone 0808 291 3363 (free, 24/7, 365 days a year)
>www.irwinmitchell.com

National Deaf Children's Society
A charity catering for deaf children and their families.

>Helpline 0808 800 8880 and SMS helpline 0786 00 22 888 (both Monday to Friday 9am–5pm)
>Email and live chat via the website www.ndcs.org.uk

Maytree Respite Centre
A registered charity supporting people in suicidal crisis in a North London non-medical setting.

>Telephone 020 7263 7070
>Email maytree@maytree.org.uk
>www.maytree.org.uk

Support for LGBTQIA+ People
Galop
A national charity supporting LGBTQIA+ people who have experienced abuse and violence.

>Domestic abuse helpline 0800 999 5428 (Monday to Friday 10am–5pm, Wednesday and Thursday 10am–8pm)
>Hate crime helpline 020 7704 2040 (Monday to Friday, 10am–4pm)
>Conversion therapy helpline 0800 130 3335 (Monday to Friday, 10am–4pm)
>Live chat via the website www.galop.org.uk

Stonewall
A national charity standing for LGBTQIA+ people everywhere and offering information, support, and advice.

>Freephone 0800 050 2020 (Monday to Friday 9.30am–4.30pm)
>Email info@stonewall.org.uk www.stonewall.org.uk

Switchboard, the LGBT+ Helpline
Switchboard provides a one-stop listening service for LGBTQIA+ people.

>Telephone 0300 330 0630 (daily 10am–10pm)
>Email chris@switchboard.lgbt
>Chat via the website www.switchboard.lgbt

Subject Index

adolescents
  atypical sexual behaviour of 71–4
  disassociation in 101–2
  talking about sex with 192
  typical sexual behaviour and development of 64–6
adult survivors
  alcohol use 129–30
  anxiety 126
  complex post-traumatic stress disorder 116–18
  depression 125
  disassociation 120–3
  drug use 129–30
  eating disorders 127
  emotional dysregulation 118–20
  intersectional issues 130–1
  memory issues 123
  mental health issues 124–5
  obsessive compulsive disorders 126–7
  personality changes 135–7
  post-traumatic stress disorder 116–18
  psychosocial impact 130
  relationship issues 137–9
  self-harm 127–8
  self-identity 134–5
  sense of self 132–3
  sexual challenges 139–41
  shame 133–4
  sleep disturbances 129
  somatisation 128–9
  suicidal thoughts/attempts 128
  therapeutic relationship 165–78
  trauma-informed practice 142–63
  triggers 124

alcohol use 129–30
anxiety 126
Assessment Intervention Moving On (AIM36) assessment 198
attachment system 102–3
atypical sexual behaviour
  in adolescents 71–4
  case illustrations for 74, 76
  and child sexual abuse 77–8
  description of 68–9
  and learning difficulties 75–7
  and neurodivergent children 74–5
  in preschool children 69–70
  in school age children 70–1
  and SSA 22–3, 78–9

Brook's Sexual Behaviours Traffic Light Tool 57–8

case illustrations
  atypical sexual behaviour 74, 76
  health warning 31–2
  impacts of SSA 82, 84, 86, 140–1
  nature of SSA 36, 38, 41–3
  risk factors in SSA 48–9, 52
  therapeutic relationships 168–70, 173–4
  trauma-informed practice 152–5, 157–8, 160–1
Child Dissociative Checklist 96
child sexual abuse
  age of perpetuators 8–9
  definition of 18–19
  prevalence of 17–18
  settings for 8

Subject Index

sexual behaviour of victims 77–8
SSA as form of 9
community-based programmes for SSA prevention 183
complex post-traumatic stress disorder (C-PTSD) 90–1, 116–18
complicity in SSA 39

definitions of SSA 18–20, 34
depression 125
developmental trauma disorder 91
Diagnostic and Statistical Manual of Mental Disorders (American Psychiatric Association) 89
disassociation 95–102, 120–3
disclosure of SSA 23–5, 144–6
drug use 129–30
'dual status' of perpetuator
  assumptions about 14–15, 19
  description of 33
  research into 195–6
  and role of professionals 25–6
dynamics of SSA 35–6

eating disorders 127
emotional dysregulation 88–9, 118–20

families
  factors in committing SSA 51–2
  interventions in 196–8
  role in SSA prevention 185

gender of perpetrators of SSA 35, 48
Good Lives Model 198
grooming process 37–9

harmful sexual behaviour (HSB)
  abuse perpetuators as victim of 14
  age of perpetrators 17
  definition of 33, 45–6
  factors in exhibiting 46–9
  family members in 33–4
  language for 31
  prevalence of 18, 46
  technology-assisted 45, 47
  and typical sexual behaviour and development 58

impacts of SSA
  alcohol use 129–30
  anxiety 126
  attachment system 102–3
  case illustrations for 82, 84, 86, 140–1
  complex post-traumatic stress disorder 90–1, 116–18
  depression 125
  developmental trauma disorder 91
  disassociation 95–102, 120–3
  drug use 129–30
  eating disorders 127
  emotional dysregulation 88–9, 118–20
  intersectional issues 130–1
  intrapersonal effects 132–41
  long-term 21–2, 115–31, 132–41
  memory issues 123
  mental health issues 124–5
  negative core beliefs 109–11
  obsessive compulsive disorders 126–7
  personality changes 135–7
  post-traumatic stress disorder 89–91, 116–18
  psychosocial impacts 130
  relational effects 132–41
  relationship issues 137–9
  self-blame 104–9
  self-harm 127–8
  self-identity 134–5
  sense of isolation 81–2
  sense of self 111–13, 132–3
  sexual challenges 139–41
  shame 104–9, 133–4
  signs of SSA 92–3
  sleep disturbances 129
  somatisation 128–9
  suicidal thoughts/attempts 128
  toxic stress 86–8
  trauma reactions 86
  triggers 124
  trust issues 104
  varieties of 84–6
Independent Inquiry into Child Sexual Abuse (IICSA) 8
International Statistical Classification of Diseases and Related Health Problems (World Health Organization) 136

intersectional issues 130–1
interventions
   in families 196–8
   with perpetuators of SSA 198–9
   with victims of SSA 199
isolation, sense of 81–2

learning difficulties 75–7

memory issues 123
mental health issues 124–5
motivations for SSA 34–5, 40–4

nature of SSA
   case illustrations for 36, 38, 41–3
   complicity in SSA 39
   dynamics of SSA 35–6
   experiences of SSA 35
   forms of 20–2
   and gender 35
   grooming process 37–9
   as HSB 33–4
   motivations for SSA 34–5, 40–4
   normalisation of SSA 36–7
   perpetuator varieties 35
   sexual behaviours in SSA 39–40
negative core beliefs 109–11
neurodivergent children 58, 74–5
normalisation of SSA 36–7, 58

obsessive compulsive disorders 126–7

personality changes 135–7
phase-orientated approach to trauma-informed practice 156–63
post-traumatic stress disorder (PTSD) 89–91, 116–18
Power Threat Meaning Framework
   professional use of 26–7, 196
   as support for survivors 16
   as trauma-informed practice 148–9
predisposing factors to commit SSA 50–5
preschool children
   atypical sexual behaviour of 69–70
   post-traumatic stress disorder in 90
   talking about sex with 188–90
   typical sexual behaviour and development of 60–2
prevalences
   of HSB 18, 46
   of sexual abuse 17–18, 46
prevention of SSA
   age-appropriate talk on sex 186–93
   community-based programmes 183
   family role in 185
   policy changes for 181
   preventative approaches to 180–1
   professional involvement in 184–5
   public education campaigns 181–5
   school-based programmes 183–4
professionals
   involvement in SSA 25–7, 196
   practice development 196
   and prevention of SSA 184–5
   in therapeutic relationship 176–7
psychosexual development 59–60
public education campaigns 181–5

relationship issues 137–9
risk factors in SSA
   case illustrations for 48–9, 52
   factors in exhibiting HSB 46–9
   family factors 51–2
   predisposing factors to commit 50–5
   prevalence of HSB 46
   socio-cultural factors 53, 54–5
school age children
   atypical sexual behaviour of 70–1
   talking about sex with 190–2
   typical sexual behaviour and development of 62–4
   school-based programmes for SSA prevention 183–4
self-blame 104–9
self-harm 127–8
self-identity 134–5
self, sense of 111–13, 132–3
sexual behaviours in SSA 39–40
sexual challenges for adult survivors 139–41
shame 104–9, 133–4, 144
sibling relationships 13–14
sibling sexual abuse (SSA)

and atypical sexual behaviour and
     development 22–3, 78–9
complexities of 15–16
definitions of 18–20, 34
disclosure of 23–5
'dual status' of perpetuator 14–15, 19
as form of child sexual abuse 9
impact of 21–2, 81–93, 95–113, 115–31
language for 31
nature of 20–2, 33–44
prevalence of 17–18
prevention of 180–93
professional involvement in 25–7
research into 195–6
risk factors in 45–56
signs of 92–3
and typical sexual behaviour
     and development 22–3
signs of SSA 92–3
sleep disturbances 129
socio-cultural factors
   in committing SSA 53, 54–5
   in typical sexual behaviour
     and development 58–9
somatisation 128–9
suicidal thoughts/attempts 128

technology-assisted HSB
     (TA-HSB) 45, 47
therapeutic relationship with
     adult survivors
   case illustrations for 168–70, 173–4
   creating secure base for 166–76

importance of 165–6
support for practitioners 176–7
toxic stress 86–8
trauma-informed practice
   case illustrations for 152–5,
     157–8, 160–1
   disclosure barriers 144–6
   phase-orientated approach 156–63
   and Power Threat Meaning
     Framework 148–9
   preparing to work with
     adult survivors 143
   principles of 149–56
   therapeutic options for 146–8
trauma reactions to SSA 86
triggers 124
trust issues 104
Truth and Repair (Herman) 157
typical sexual behaviour
     and development
   in adolescents 64–6
   and Brook's Sexual Behaviours
     Traffic Light Tool 57–8
   and HSB 58
   and learning difficulties 75–7
   and neurodivergent children 58,
     74–5
   and normalisation of SSA 58
   in preschool children 60–2
   psychosexual development in 59–60
   in school age children 62–4
   and SSA 22–3
   socio-cultural factors in 58–9

Author Index

Adler, N.A. 36, 52
Adshead, G. 169, 174
Albanese, M.J. 129
Allardyce, S. 9, 13, 17, 18, 19, 20, 21, 23, 24, 25, 26, 31, 34, 35, 43, 46, 47, 51, 54, 116, 185, 196, 197, 199
American Psychiatric Association 82, 89, 91, 116
Atwood, J.D. 18, 34

Baldwin, J.D. 60
Baldwin, J.I. 60
Bales, S.N. 86
Ballantine, M.W. 21, 85
Baranowsky, A. 145, 147, 156
Barra, S. 46
Beckett, R. 18, 34
Belton, E. 45
Bentovim, A. 47
Berger, R. 149
Blokland, A. 31
Blue Beat Studios 192
Boon, S. 122
Bovarnick, S. 185
Bowlby, J. 112
Boyle, M. 16, 26, 30, 136, 142, 148, 196, 198
Buie, D.H. 172
Butler, L.D. 149

Caffaro, J. 18, 22, 23, 24, 34, 35, 50, 52, 54, 82, 103, 116, 181, 183, 184, 198, 199
Campbell, S.M. 198
Canavan, M.M. 40, 52
Caretti, V. 97, 111

Carlson, B.E. 35, 40
Caspi, J. 19, 43
Children's Commissioner for England 8
Choi, K.R. 101, 102
Cloitre, M. 159
Cohen, J.A. 89
Conn-Caffaro, A. 18, 23, 34, 35, 50, 82, 103
Courtois, C.A. 50, 103, 145, 147, 156, 159, 196
Cozolino, L. 166
Cundy, L. 47
Cyr, M. 50

De Jong, A.R. 35
Dearing, R.L. 106
Department of Education 18–19
Department of Health 54
DiGiorgio-Miller, J. 35

Elliott, D.E. 149
Enns, C.Z. 21
Erooga, M. 46

Fallot, R.D. 149
Felitti, V.J. 129
Finkelhor, D. 18, 34, 35, 103
Fisher, J. 122
Fonagy, P. 169, 174
Ford, J.D. 50, 103, 145, 147, 156, 159, 196
Forgash, C. 146
Friedrich, W. 18, 47

Author Index

Gelinas, D.J. 146
Gentry, J.E. 145, 147, 156
Glaser, D. 19, 43
Griffee, K. 52

Hackett, S. 18, 31, 33, 34, 45, 46, 47, 180, 184, 185, 198, 199
Hamama, L. 21
Hardy, M.S. 18, 34, 52
Harris, M. 149
Herman, J. 136, 145, 147, 156, 157, 159, 163
Hollis, V. 45
Howell, E.F. 112
Hughes, C. 13

International Society for the Study of Trauma and Dissociation 99
Israel, E. 52

Jay, A. 8
Johnson, T. 78
Johnstone, L. 16, 26, 30, 136, 142, 148, 196, 198
Jordan, J.V. 156, 170, 171, 175

Katz, C. 21
Kelly, L. 54
Khantzian, E.J. 129
Knipe, J. 146
Krienert, J.L. 18, 34

Lanius, R.A. 96
Latzman, N.E. 34, 52
Laviola, M. 35
Letourneau, E.J. 180
Levine, P.A. 146, 160
Lewis, H.B. 106, 107
Loredo, C. 52
Lussier, P. 31, 46

Maltsberger, J.T. 172
Masson, H. 46, 198
Maté, G. 129
McCartan, K. 19, 20, 21, 22, 23, 24, 25, 26, 27, 34, 35, 43, 48, 51, 53, 54, 82, 116, 181, 196, 197, 199

McKillop, N. 31, 46
McNeish, D. 31, 46, 47
Mead, D. 47
Mercer, J. 199
Miller, J.B. 156, 170, 171, 175
Mollon, P. 112
Myers, I.J. 103

Najavits, L. 149
Nathanson, D.L. 108
NSPCC 45, 54

O'Brien, M.J. 34, 35
Ogden, P. 146, 160
O'Keefe, S.L. 23, 35
One in Four 129, 134

Payne, P. 146, 160
Pearlman, L.A. 177
Perry, B.D. 95, 96, 102
Punch, S. 13
Putnam, F.W. 95

Quiros, L. 149

Rothschild, B. 147, 156, 160, 172, 173
Ryan, G. 47
Rydberg, J.A. 160

Saakvitne, K.W. 177
Sabina, C. 47
Sanderson, C. 17, 25, 26, 39, 54, 59, 61, 82, 85, 86, 100, 103, 104, 106, 107, 108, 109, 116, 118, 123, 127, 129, 134, 137, 139, 143, 144, 145, 146, 147, 148, 150, 151, 153, 156, 158, 160, 162, 163, 165, 166, 170, 171, 172, 173, 175, 176, 178, 186, 188, 189, 196
Saunders, B. 198
Scheeringa, M.S. 82, 89
Schimmenti, A. 97, 111
Schutz, J. 35, 52
Scott, S. 31, 46, 47, 185
Shah, R.S. 54
Shapiro, E. 146
Sharpe, M. 47
Shaw, J.A. 18, 34

Shonkoff, J.P. 86
Skovholt, T.M. 178
Smith, C. 180, 185
Smith, H. 52
Stathopoulos, M. 19
Steele, K. 122, 146
Stermac, L.E. 19, 43
Stripe, T.S. 19, 43
Stroebel, S.S. 18, 34, 35, 50, 103

Tangney, J.P. 106
Tener, D. 18, 199
Tidefors, I. 34, 52
Tougas, A.M. 46
Trotter-Mathison, M. 178
Turner, H.A. 185
Twombly, J.H. 146

Van der Hart, O. 98, 99, 122, 146
Van der Kolk, B. 86, 91, 129, 147, 156, 158, 160
Veale, D. 111
Vizard, E. 46

Walsh, J.A. 18, 34
Ward, T. 198
White, N. 13
Wiehe, V.R. 18, 19, 34, 43
Wissink, I.B. 54
World Health Organization 91, 116, 136
Worling, J.R. 52

Yates P. 9, 13, 17, 18, 19, 20, 21, 23, 24, 25, 26, 31, 34, 35, 43, 46, 47, 51, 52, 54, 58, 116, 185, 196, 197, 199